AF443247

# A B C OF OPHTHALMOLOGY

# A B C OF OPHTHALMOLOGY

P A GARDINER

Articles published in
the *British Medical Journal*

Published by the British Medical Association
Tavistock Square, London WC1H 9JR

First Edition April 1979
Reprinted December 1979
Reprinted October 1981

Made and printed in England by
The Devonshire Press
Barton Road, Torquay

# Preface

by the Editor
*British Medical Journal*

Few doctors learn much about ophthalmology while at medical school, yet visual problems are common in medical practice and are often a sign of more generalised disease.

We have recently published a series of straightforward articles by Mr P A Gardiner on the visual problems that a general practitioner might see in his surgery. All the common problems are covered—squints, glaucoma, cataracts—together with instruction on examination, diagnosis, and management and an account of the services available for visually handicapped people.

These articles are collected together here to provide quick practical guidance on eye conditions and help in assessing priorities in treatment. We hope that they will serve their purpose.

STEPHEN LOCK
1979

# Contents

# ACCIDENTS AND FIRST AID

## Assess acuity in both eyes

Urgent treatment

Assess acuity in
both eyes

Do not use local
anaesthetics for
treatment

Trauma to the eye clearly needs urgent treatment. Equally important is the fact that even a trivial injury to the only good eye of a pair is potentially far more serious than it would be if both eyes have good equal acuity.

The acuity of the uninjured eye is far more important at the outset than that of the injured eye because it indicates the level of care that is needed, perhaps making all the difference between admission or outpatient treatment. The acuity should be recorded in all cases, for both clinical and medicolegal reasons.

As a general principle local anaesthetics should not be used more than once, though general sedation is often sensible. Atropine drops 1% or mydrilate, which dilate the pupil, often give great relief from pain.

## Chemical and thermal burns: immediate first aid

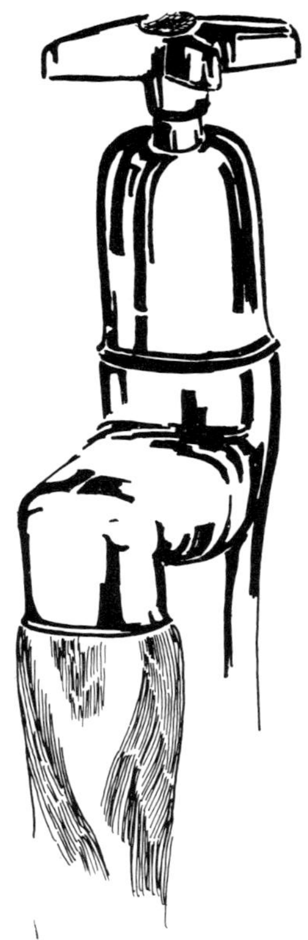

Immediate first aid is needed in all forms of chemical burns. Speed is essential, and the eyes should be washed out with copious amounts of any clean water. This may be difficult because pain causes spasm of the lids, but it must be attempted, and within seconds if possible.

Many chemical burns have late complications, notably lime burns because of retained particles. Therefore all burns that affect the globe require early hospital attention. Late complications include adhesions of the globe to the lid, so that liberal and frequent applications of chloramphenicol ointment or drops are desirable.

It is difficult to know whether to cover the eye, but the retention of toxic substances and danger of adhesions will be less if the eye remains uncovered or only loosely covered.

In many corneal conditions extremely painful iris spasm may often occur. This is indicated by constriction of the pupil, but even without this sign the patient is likely to be much more comfortable if mydrilate 1% or atropine 1% is instilled. Dark glasses are helpful.

Many chemicals have specific antidotes, but searching for these may cause delay. A supply of antidotes is clearly necessary in industrial practice, where there may be particular risks from specific toxic agents. The antidote to lime, for example, is a saturated solution of glucose.

# Accidents and first aid

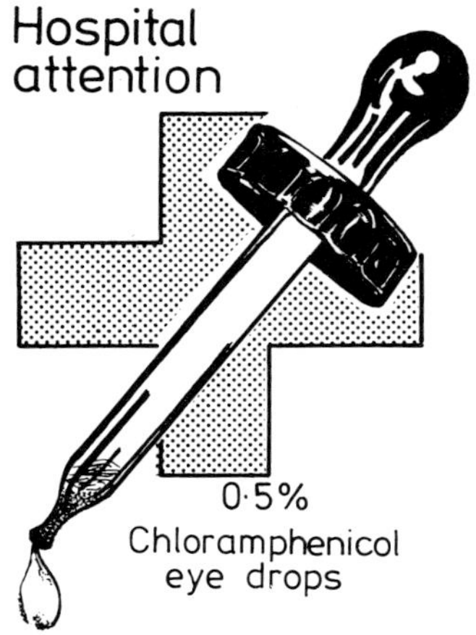



Thermal burns seldom affect only the globe, but general sedation and an antibiotic drop or ointment into the eye is sensible treatment.

When only the lids are injured externally the ultimate dangers are less and less immediate. Burnt lids should be treated like any other burn of the skin, though eventually scarring in more severe cases may lead to complications affecting the globe.

## Sharp wounds: general management

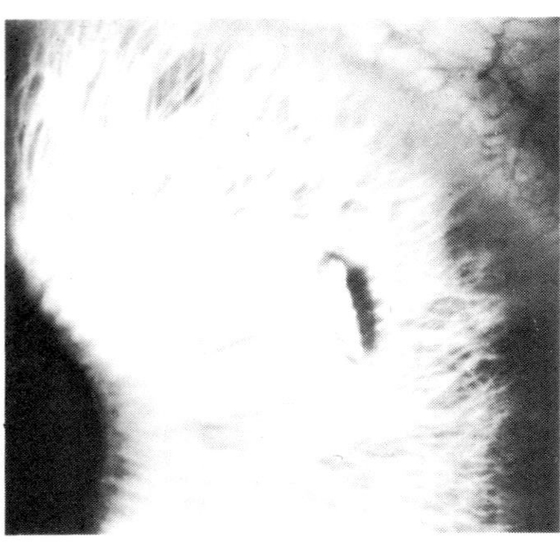

When serious damage of the eye is feared the less examination of the eye that is carried out the better. If the globe is likely to have been damaged attempts to determine the extent of the wound may extend the damage. The patient should be immobilised, given a general analgesic if he is in severe pain, and transferred rapidly to the casualty department of a hospital that has facilities for eye surgery. No pressure should be put on the eye, so any covering should be light.

Penetrating wounds, which are often surprisingly painless, need urgent attention because the longer repair is delayed the more danger there is of the intraocular contents being disturbed or extruded and the greater the chance of infection.

## Penetrating wounds: state of pupil an important sign

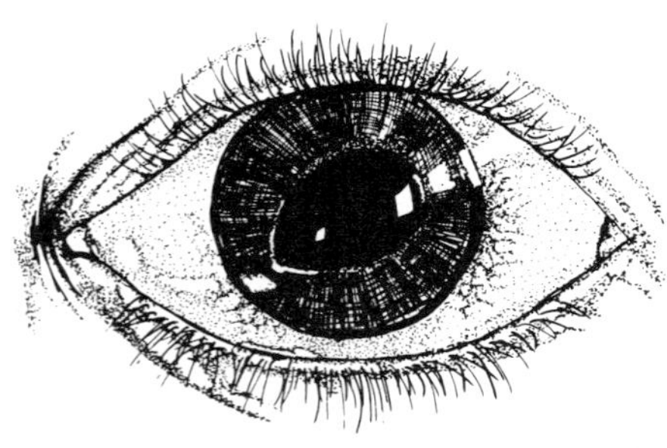

An important sign of penetration is the state of the pupil. Instillation of a local anaesthetic, such as amethocaine, may be necessary to make this examination, which is harmless in a co-operative patient. The use of such an anaesthetic should not be continued to relieve pain, however, as it may delay healing or promote further damage. A penetrating wound is usually indicated by a deformed (oval) and sluggish pupil. If the pupil is deformed, however slight other signs may be, penetration must be assumed until it has been definitely excluded. Nevertheless, a round pupil does not indicate that penetration has not occurred.

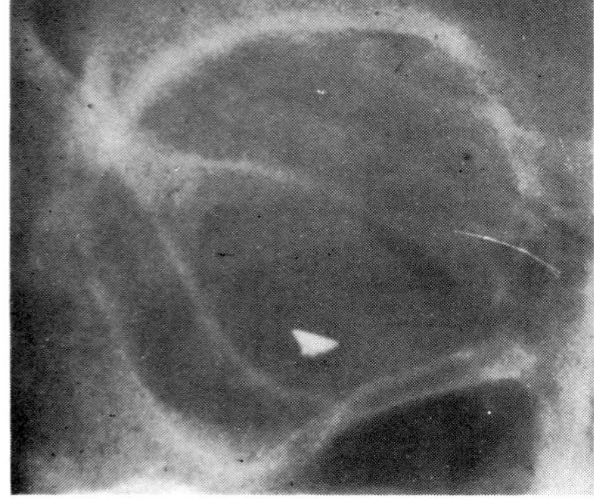

Injuries from flying particles, during operations such as grinding or chipping with hammer and chisel, are particularly misleading. In grinding, high-velocity metal particles may penetrate the eye and eventually lead to blindness with little or no apparent external injury or pain. In chipping it is often falsely assumed that a fragment from the object being chiselled has entered the eye, whereas it is just as common for a particle from one of the tools to have done so. It is important to find a foreign body in these cases and essential to take an *x*-ray picture. Retained intraocular foreign bodies may cause blindness many years later.

# Removing foreign bodies: harder than it looks

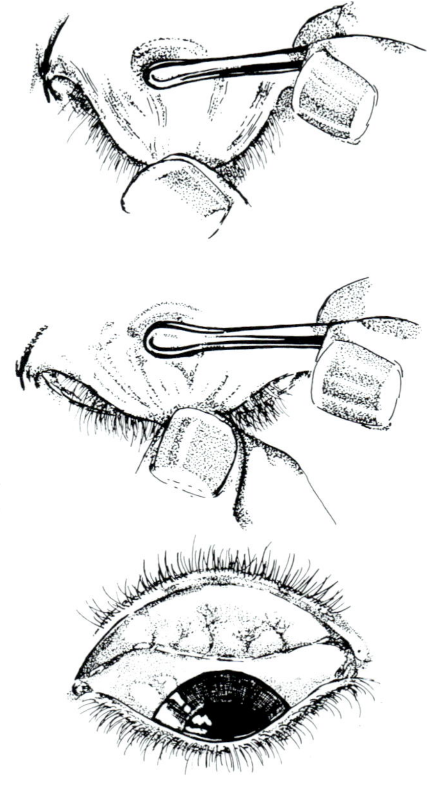

The pain in superficial wounds may be much greater than with penetrating wounds, especially if the cornea is affected. Superficial foreign bodies are most often found either inside the upper or lower lid or on the cornea. The sensation of a foreign body under the lid, scraping the cornea with each blink, is identical with that of a scratch on the cornea without a foreign body. A good search for a foreign body and its removal in the surgery will spare the patient a visit to hospital. A local anaesthetic is usually needed.

Most foreign bodies look black against the lid or sclera but are often difficult to identify against the background of the iris or the pupil. A drop of fluorescein dye will help to identify the lesion through washing round a corneal foreign body or staining a corneal abrasion. It is difficult to find quite large foreign bodies under the upper lid without exposing the inner surface of the lid, which is often impossible, even under local anaesthesia. If it proves impossible the patient should be referred to an ophthalmologist if the symptoms or history of a foreign body are present.

Removing a foreign body from the lower lid is comparatively easy if the patient is co-operative. The patient's head should be firmly supported, and a local anaesthetic (amethocaine 1%) should be given if the foreign body is on the cornea. It may also be helpful if the foreign body is under the lids.

A good instrument to use in removing a foreign body is a piece of white postcard cut into a triangular shape. Gripped by one angle of the triangle the opposing sharp point will remove all superficial foreign bodies with far less trauma than a metallic instrument, especially if the particle has to be pursued across the eye after it is loosened.

Any foreign bodies that resist this technique need more expert removal with more dangerous instruments. Removal should be followed by immediate instillation of an antibiotic (chloramphenicol), as the procedure is not sterile. If the cornea has been affected it is wise to pad the eye for about two hours or longer if the pain returns. A bright light, self-retaining lid speculum, and magnification are all aids. Follow-up is advisable if the affected eye is the only useful one, and whenever possible acuity should be recorded in both eyes before treatment and in the injured eye after healing.

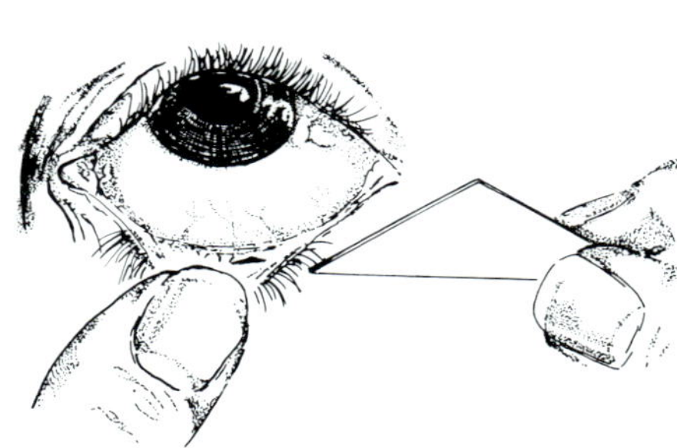

# Corneal abrasions

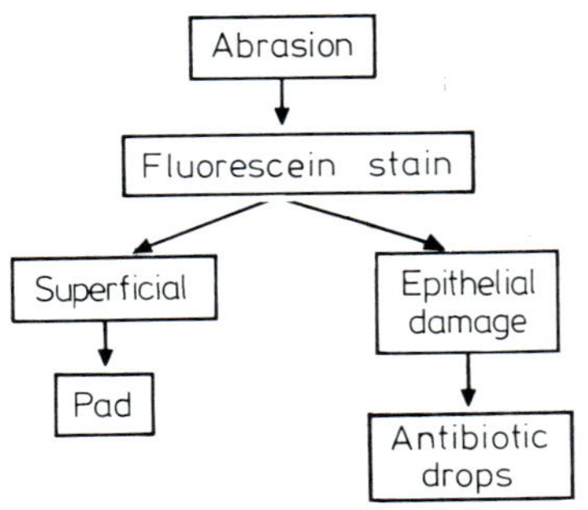


Scratches on the cornea commonly accompany foreign bodies and attempts at their removal. At home a baby's fingernail, or in the garden stakes and twigs, are most to be feared. All abrasions stain with fluorescein. Superficial corneal abrasions heal quickly in about 48 hours with a firm pad to stop blinking and therefore reactivation of the damage; preventing blinking also has an analgesic effect. Local anaesthesia delays healing but dilating the pupil also relieves pain. In all cases when fluorescein staining indicates epithelial damage antibiotic drops twice a day should be used until healing has occurred. Persistence of an abrasion or pain beyond 48 hours may well indicate complications.

# Blunt injuries: test acuity and exclude internal haemorrhage

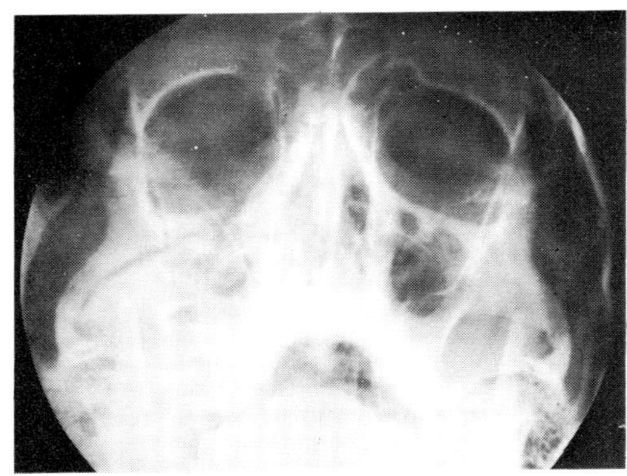

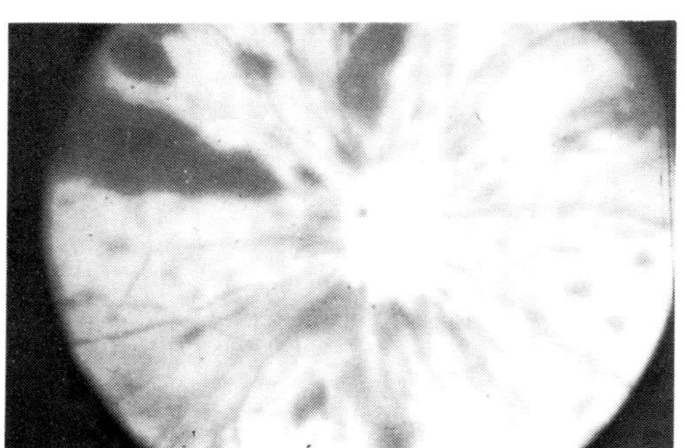

Blunt injuries are characterised by the familiar black eye, which is caused by impact with objects larger than the orbit. The visual damage is unlikely to be as bad as external appearances suggest. The commonest complication of these injuries is double vision, which needs to be tested for at the full range of vision as soon as the eye is open.

Recovery tends to be spontaneous except when the orbital wall is fractured. Then urgent treatment is needed to reconstitute the normal bony structure, which will prevent permanent limitation of movement caused by secondary adhesions or fibrosis of the extraocular muscles. Relief from diplopia may always be obtained by covering one eye, though at the expense of depth perception in patients with previously good binocular vision.

Ocular effects include haemorrhage into all parts of the globe: intraocular haemorrhages will obviously usually diminish visual acuity. Such haemorrhages need differentiation by an ophthalmologist, and physical rest is sensible until their nature and source has been established. Later complications include secondary retinal detachment. In most cases it is sensible to instil mydrilate two or three times a day until the absence of intraocular damage is proved.

The most dangerous injuries apart from those caused by traffic accidents are those caused by shotgun and airgun pellets, squash balls and champagne corks—projectiles that are small in relation to the orbit. Fireworks and all games with bows and arrows are dangerous to children. Such incidents are largely preventable by good discipline. Certain types of swimming goggles can cause dangerous injuries.

A dilated paralysed pupil is often the only sign of a blunt injury. This usually recovers in days or weeks but is often associated with haemorrhage into the vitreous, which must be excluded in every case.

# Burns from sun and snow

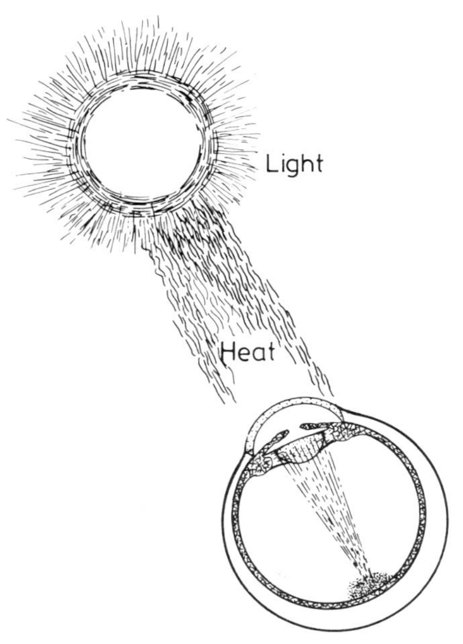


Like its light rays the sun's heat rays are focused on the retina. Intense light initiates a defence mechanism to protect the retina by closing the eyes. Children who have competed with each other to see who could keep their eyes open longest while looking straight at the sun have often burnt their retinas and suffered a considerable permanent loss of vision. This is a variety of the eclipse blindness produced by watching the sun in eclipse with unprotected eyes, when focusing of the heat rays is not prevented by a response to the sun's light. In sleep the retina is protected by the globe rolling upwards into the orbit. Ambient sunlight is harmless in Britain.

Ultraviolet radiation in the so-called "arc eye" or in snow blindness may cause extremely distressing superficial effects some time after exposure and occurs if the eyes are not protected by tinted shields. Danger to sight is, however, minimal. Emergency treatment is of little avail, though bandaging with cold compresses gives partial relief of the pain, and adrenaline drops will reduce congestion temporarily. The use of amethocaine is justified, and its effects are sometimes dramatic. Atropine drops are useful if the pupils are painfully constricted as they reduce the element of spasm.

The photographs of an intraocular foreign body and intraocular haemorrhage were reproduced by permission of the Institute of Ophthalmology. The radiographs of an intraocular foreign body and orbital fracture were reproduced from *System of Ophthalmology* edited by Sir Stewart Duke-Elder vol 14, part I by kind permission of the publishers, Henry Kimpton Ltd.

# MANAGEMENT OF DEFECTS OF VISION IN EARLY CHILDHOOD

## Developing the brain

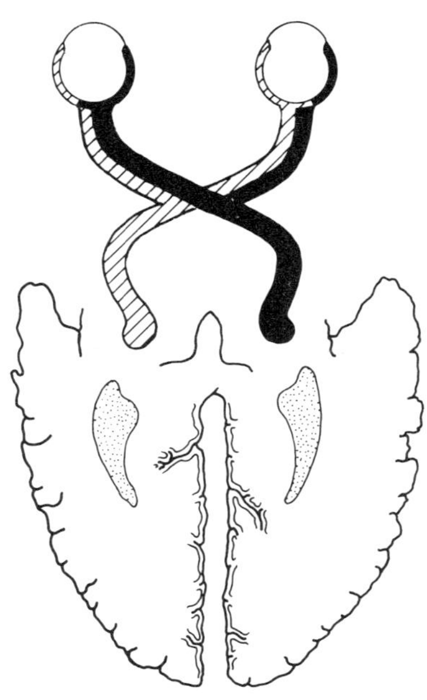

At birth both the retina and the occipital cortex are incomplete. Development of these elements depends on use, so correct vision is important in childhood. If the eye receives no stimulus vision will be impaired and the actual apparatus for seeing will not become fully developed.

Vision therefore has to be learnt by degrees at the proper time, one vital period being infancy. Thus a child with congenital cataracts must have surgery early to avoid a permanent and irreversible visual defect, which would occur if surgery were delayed much beyond the first year.

Babies are interested in their fingers or blanket threads or crumbs from a very young age but do not become interested in more distant events until they leave their cots and become mobile. Visual experience therefore seems to be acquired first from near objects and later from distant ones.

The infant builds up a framework of visual information that is secure for near objects before venturing into the space beyond. It is much harder to establish a relationship with distant areas, possibly because of the sheer number of visual impressions that need analysis—movement and colour being added problems. Judging distances, for example, requires much experience and experiment.

## Action to establish normality of vision

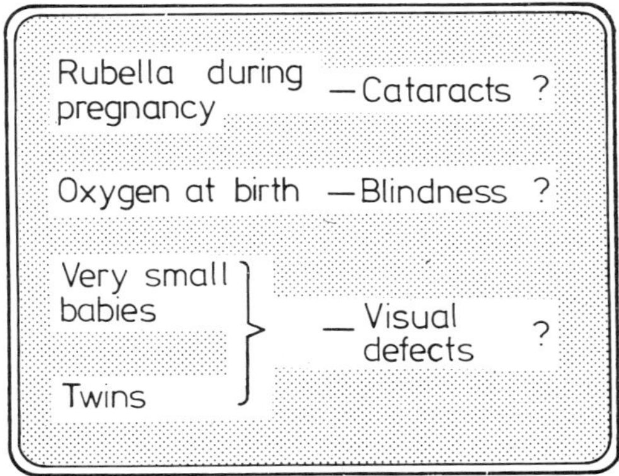


Therefore a system for detecting defects is needed. Children who are learning all the time will not complain about a visual defect until they can make valid comparisons with their fellows. This often does not happen until about the age of 10, but by then they will often suppress the knowledge of their defect for fear of the treatment.

Ideally every infant's acuity should be tested in infant welfare and developmental clinics. When time or skill is short particular attention should be paid to certain groups.

Antenatal and perinatal influences may have important effects on vision. For example, rubella in the first three months of pregnancy may cause cataracts in an infant. Oxygen given at birth may blind or seriously impair vision. Very small babies have a greater risk of eye defects than others, as do twins.

# Management of defects of vision in early childhood

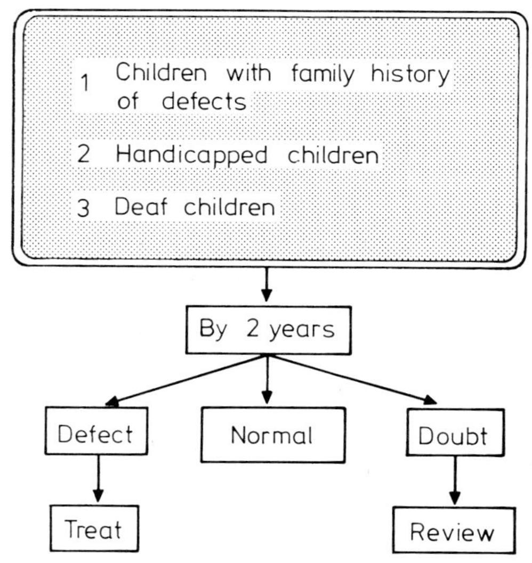



Children with any physical or mental handicap—particularly the brain-damaged—are likely to have more than one handicap, and this may be visual. Another special group are the deaf, who although they are not especially likely to have visual defects, do need a higher visual standard earlier than other children if they are not to be at a disadvantage in lip reading and interpreting the moods of others by vision rather than tone of voice. Infants whose close relatives had defects from infancy also need special examination.

In all these groups positive action to establish the normality of vision is essential and can be carried out in infant assessment centres. Doctors should not be satisfied by negative results but should seek specialist help if any doubt arises. By the age of 2 visual performance in these groups should have been correctly assessed and any necessary treatment started. In many children doubt will remain and continuing regular assessments need to be made.

## Family history and hereditary disorders

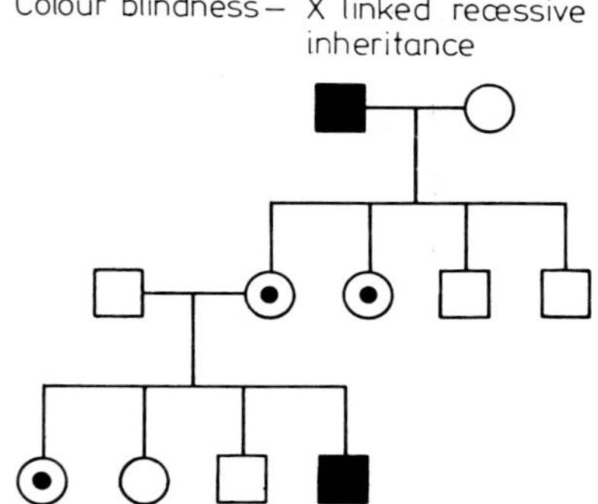



Hereditary visual disorders will generally manifest themselves at the same age in each generation. It is therefore senseless to look for glaucoma in an infant because many relatives became glaucomatous in middle age. It is also a misconception that myopic parents will produce short-sighted babies unless they themselves were born short-sighted. If the parents became myopic later in childhood, however, then their children are likely to repeat this pattern.

## Severe refractive disorders

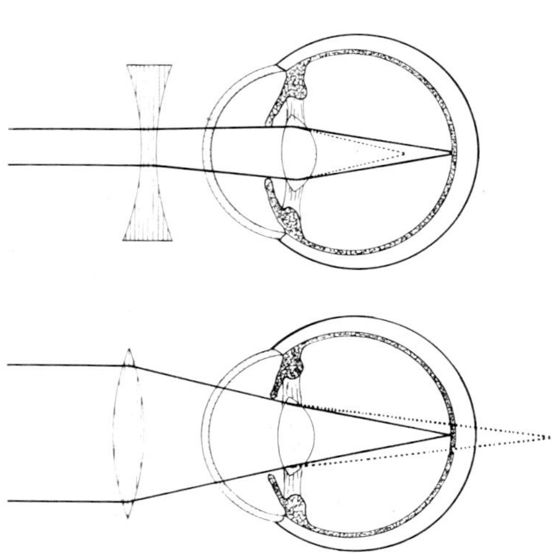

Congenital disorders of refraction, whether long sight or astigmatism, appear to be inherited conditions. If they are very severe in the parent they should be looked for in early childhood. Mild refractive anomalies are not important to infant development, but severe forms may be. This is particularly true of severe hypermetropia, which predisposes to the appearance of squints or to the neglect of one eye. Once refraction has been performed and an anomaly identified it is a matter of judgment precisely when to order glasses.

Despite the growth of the eye, any optical anomaly will alter very little except in those who acquire myopia during later childhood.

As well as establishing the transparency of the eye and presence of a normal retina, any ophthalmological investigations must include an assessment of refraction. Severely abnormal acuity may have a profound effect on visual development. Glasses must be provided even at very early ages.

When screening among children was not performed it was common to see adults severely short-sighted from birth or later who had never worn glasses. When given glasses these improved their sight only slightly. Often the extra amount of vision proved an intolerable amount of visual information and the glasses were discarded. This state of affairs is preventable only by finding and treating defects as soon as they arise in childhood.

# Management of defects of vision in early childhood

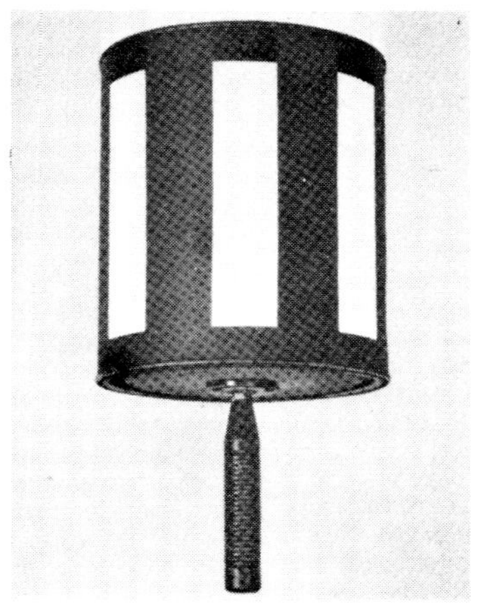

Short-sighted children benefit immediately from glasses. Their unaided good near vision will have provided them with a background of partial visual education that the highly long-sighted child does not possess. The long-sighted child will therefore have to learn to interpret the new images that glasses provide him with before deriving the greatest benefit.

The tests available up to the age of 3 are cumbersome, time consuming, and often inconclusive. So further investigation is needed by an ophthalmologist in the children in the groups at risk who do not carry them out convincingly. These tests include those based on opticokinetic nystagmus, unmasking balls of varying diameters, and matching tests. Test failures should never be expressed confidently as a visual defect in the absence of an ophthalmological examination because it is so often due to a lack of concentration rather than to visual failure.

## Simple tests of vision

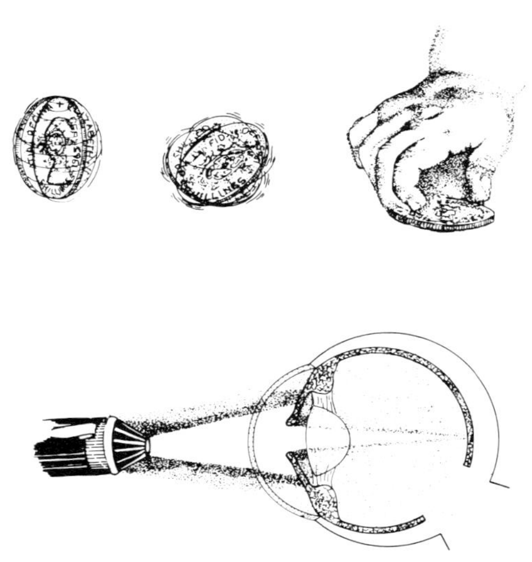

The place and technique of testing visual acuity must depend on the level of accuracy that is being aimed at. Thus a paediatric assessment centre will need the whole panoply of apparatus. There are, however, several useful but non-complex methods that can be used in ordinary surroundings so that a health visitor (for example) can make some judgment on the need for further advice. These include spinning a coin; this should attract a child's attention, but the crucial moment is when the coin falls silent. If the child moves to pick it up it is evidence of useful vision and that he was not just responding to the noise. Another important piece of evidence is if a child turns his eyes towards a torch, but beware of the click of the switch being heard. Small sweets such as Smarties and, even better, "hundreds and thousands" are also useful in testing a young child's ability to see.

The most reliable simple test of basic ocular function is the pupil's reaction to light. If this is present in an infant who is otherwise normal then the outlook for useful vision is good, however unresponsive to other tests he may be.

## School entry: greater demand on eyesight

| 2 years | No gross defect ? |
|---------|-------------------|
| 5 years | Test: Distance vision, Near vision, Colour vision |
| >5 years | Myopia ? |

The increasing development of skills and mobility makes more demands on eyesight the older the child grows. Formal screening of visual acuity at school entry is therefore essential. This test is necessary not only on general grounds but also to ensure that education is not retarded. It is wise to include a test for near vision as well as distant vision, because impaired near vision will increase fatigue and indicates hypermetropia or astigmatism.

The examination at school entry should include a simple test for colour vision defects in boys. About 10% of boys have difficulty with colour discrimination and about 5% have a considerable hereditary red-green deficiency. Any defect remains unchanged through life but it seems sensible to identify it as early as possible.

Colour blindness is so rare as to be of little importance, but defects in discrimination can catch out and distress young children who are unaware of their defect.

It should be established before the age of 2 that there is no gross defect in sight and by 5 that both distance and near vision are adequate in each eye if not perfect. After 5 deterioration in the absence of disease is not likely to occur except in the 10-15% of children destined to become short-sighted in middle or late childhood.

The photograph of the opticokinetic nystagmus drum is reproduced by kind permission of Keeler Instruments Ltd.

# SQUINTS

## Looking at different things

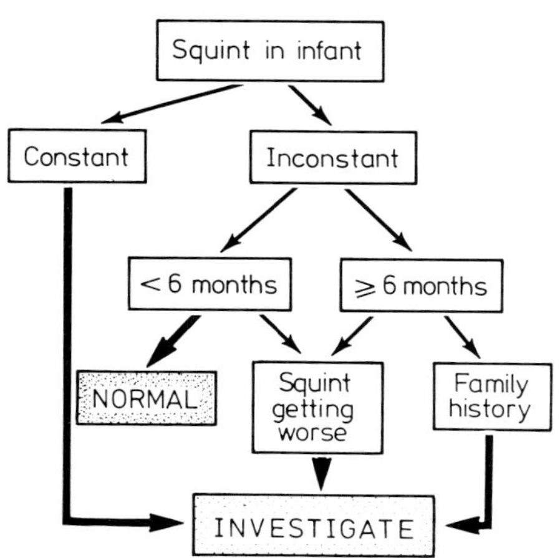

In a squinting child the two eyes do not look at the same thing. Squints first show themselves in the years when eyesight and its use are developing, so they may easily be thought to affect the eyesight in some way. But such is the power of adaptation in children and young infants that if each eye is used alternately visual acuity is not affected.

Squints may be divided into those that are constantly present and those that are present only at times; those that are confined to one eye and those that affect each eye at different times. These distinctions are important. A child who has a constant squint in one eye cannot have normal sight in that eye. If there is a constant squint that affects each eye alternately the vision is usually equal in each eye and often completely normal.

A constant squint, especially in the early weeks of life, demands immediate full investigation to exclude local or general disease. An inconstant squint is another matter. Until a baby has learnt to look at an object inconstant squints are very common. Inconstant squints that persist after the age of 6 months demand ophthalmological assessment if there is a family history of early squinting or if one eye seems to be squinting more frequently than the other or the squint is becoming more common or lasting longer.

## Binocular vision

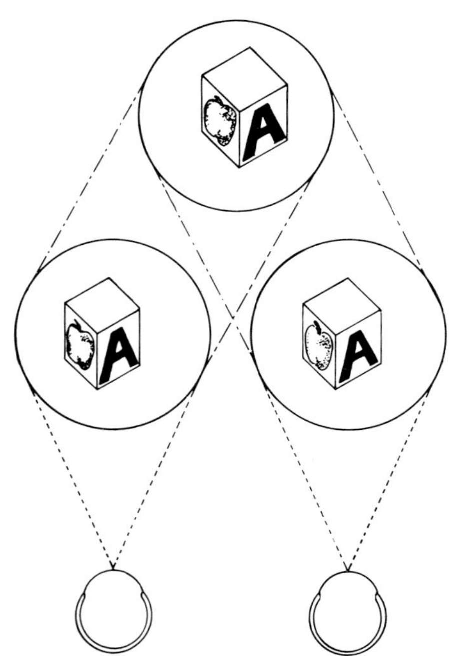

Children who constantly squint cannot develop true binocular vision. This has little importance in daily life because of the infant's ability to adapt. Adults who lose the use of one eye have great difficulty in judging depth and distance, but children adapt quickly and compensate fully. This ability to adapt diminishes progressively after about the age of 7.

Adults who begin to squint also have double vision, whereas most children who squint, especially those with constant squints, tend not to. Those children with inconstant squints who do see double nevertheless adapt very well. Adults who grew up with well-compensated double vision have driven fast cars and assisted at surgical operations with no difficulty.

Unlike the adult, the child is both learning to see objects of importance and learning not to see confusing images. If he has a constant squint in only one eye he will suppress double vision by permanently disregarding the image from this eye—at the cost of losing a great deal of acuity. If the squint is alternating from eye to eye he will disregard the image of each eye temporarily. In the first case only one eye will develop normal eyesight, whereas in the other both will see normally. Common sense seems to indicate that a squint in both eyes must be worse than in only one. This is wrong.

# Diagnosing squints: cosmetic judgments misleading

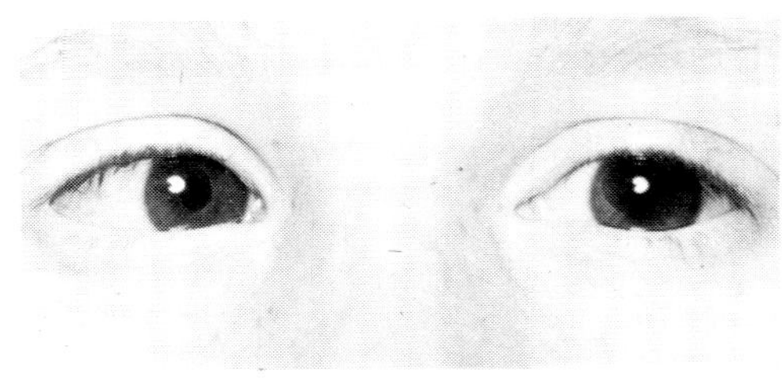

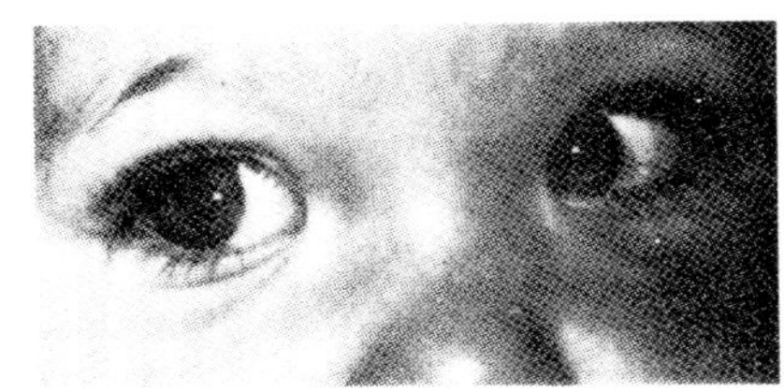

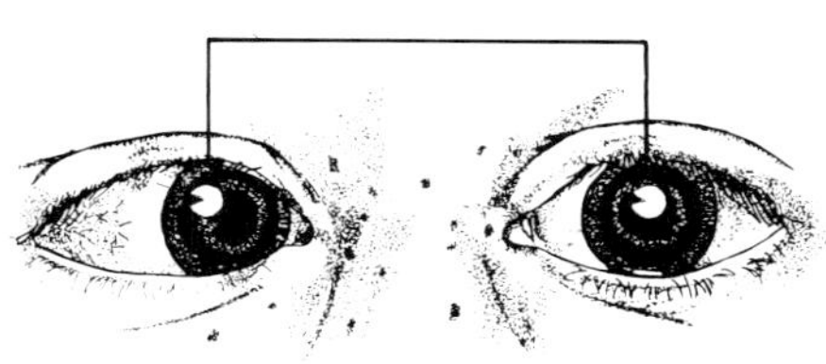

The effects of squints on acuity are hidden because the child is unaware of the peculiarity, so most judgments on squints are cosmetic. These are often misleading. A small-angle squint may go unnoticed but its effect on visual acuity might be just as serious as that of a squint that is offensive to look at. Alternating squints are often misjudged in this way because they are often very obvious, but the visual acuity in each eye may be equal and normal.

The difficulty in noticing small-angle squints, which causes delay in treatment, indicates the need to search actively for them. Treatment should be started as soon as possible, before the child loses his adaptive abilities, and preferably before compensatory mechanisms become established and have to be unlearnt. Infant welfare clinics and the community eye services can perform a valuable role in screening children for these defects.

A common source of misdiagnosis is the fold of skin at the inner angle of each eye in infants who have a wide or no bridge to their nose. This epicanthic fold hides some of the nasal portion of the globe, producing the illusion of a squint in perfectly straight eyes.

Squints may be difficult to diagnose, especially in infancy, when the diagnosis is most important. It should be possible to observe the dissimilar positions of light reflected from each eye that occurs in a squint, but only if the infant is co-operative and interested and actually fixing a target. Such infants are rare. First covering one eye and then the other should produce movement in a squinting eye but not in a straight eye. But again the infant's co-operation and interest are essential, and even then it is difficult to be sure that the movements of the eye are produced because of the squint and not spontaneously.

Though horizontal squints are the most common, a vertical element may be present and may show itself by the child tilting his head to compensate. This important diagnostic guide is often overlooked and attributed to abnormal neck muscles.

# Treatment: glasses, patching, and surgery

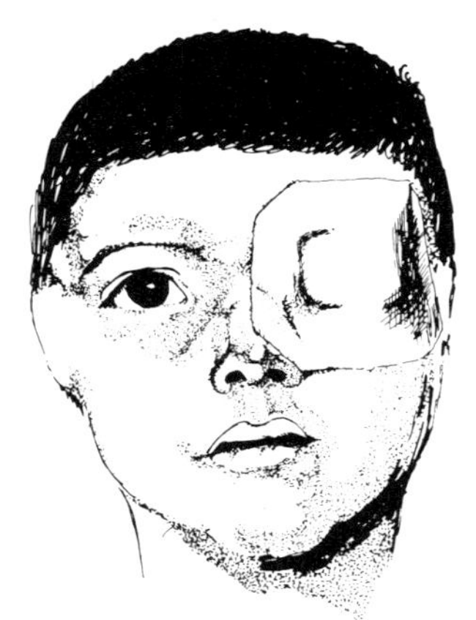


The aims of treatment are: (1) to eliminate defects of visual acuity; (2) to achieve a satisfactory appearance; and (3) to arrive at good binocular vision. The last is the ultimate aim, but it is seldom achieved; its pursuit is tedious, and failure is not a grave handicap. Parents should be reassured about this.

The treatment of the visual defect is the most important element of treatment. Disuse of an eye prevents the development of its vision, and treatment is aimed at making the eye work. This demands spectacles, patching, and surgery.

Glasses not only provide the correct optical situation for normal vision; they also eliminate the effort, subconscious though it may be, of focusing images, which in many young children is the real cause of a squint. Many squints are rectified by the use of glasses alone, even those where visual acuity is good.

Patching compels the defective eye to take up the load that it is normally disinclined to bear, because of either its angle or its optical burden. Acuity in the defective eye may take weeks to match that in the better eye, or it may never happen. Ideally, once the acuity of the defective eye has improved to equal that of its partner surgery should be performed.

In theory the child then begins anew with straight eyes, which are equal in vision. Cosmetically, the eye will usually appear satisfactory, though several operations may be needed. In many cases, however, the originally defective eye will still have less effective vision, or it may relapse in terms of acuity.

## Surgery as insurance

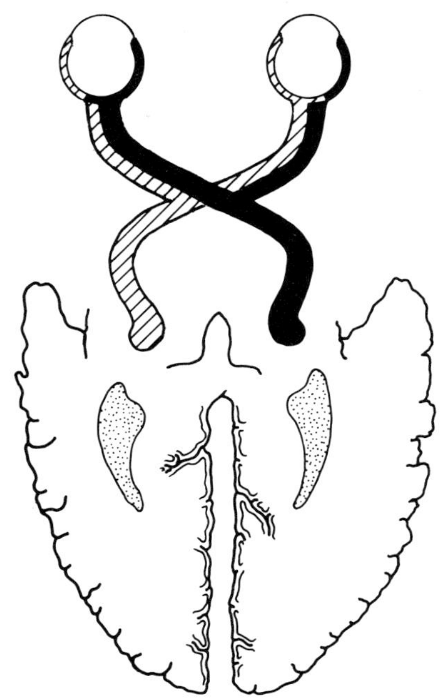

Nevertheless, surgery for squints is technically simple and not a great demand on healthy children, and the cosmetic improvement is of great benefit psychologically.

Also treatment has achieved much as an insurance. Once an eye has been made to see and the cortex has practised interpreting its activities, it is a potentially useful eye, even though it may relapse. Should the other eye fail through injury or disease, the treated eye can take over. If no attempt is made in early childhood to improve acuity in a constantly squinting eye, then its owner is permanently equipped with only one useful eye. This may be a psychological handicap, even though it may not be a visual one.

It is often difficult to explain to parents that an operation for squint may have no effect on vision, yet any delay may cause loss of the opportunity to develop good vision in the squinting eye. The child's reactions to treatment are also important. For example, occluding the good eye may severely handicap a child, producing blurring that may be profoundly disturbing.

Children who are particularly likely to be disturbed by treatment (including surgery) are those with other handicaps. Late walkers, late talkers, and so on may revert to an earlier stage, losing painfully won ground by injudicious treatment for a squint. In such cases close co-operation between all the doctors looking after the child is therefore important.

## Balancing the benefits and drawbacks

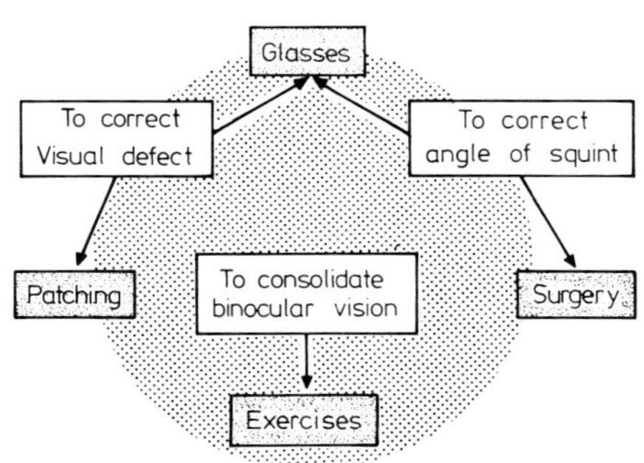


The programme for treatment of squints can therefore be summarised as correction of the visual defect by glasses or patching or both; correction of the angle by surgery or glasses or both; and consolidation of any binocular vision by exercises under an orthoptist. Treatment should be started within weeks of a squint being noticed and should be completed by the age of 7. After this the prospect of any improvement except a cosmetic one becomes less and less likely.

Fewer than half the children treated for squint gain the benefit of having two eyes with really good acuity and good binocular vision. A crippling treatment (and its duration) must be balanced against the ultimate gain. It is seldom of any use to begin patching after the age of 6.

## Amblyopia

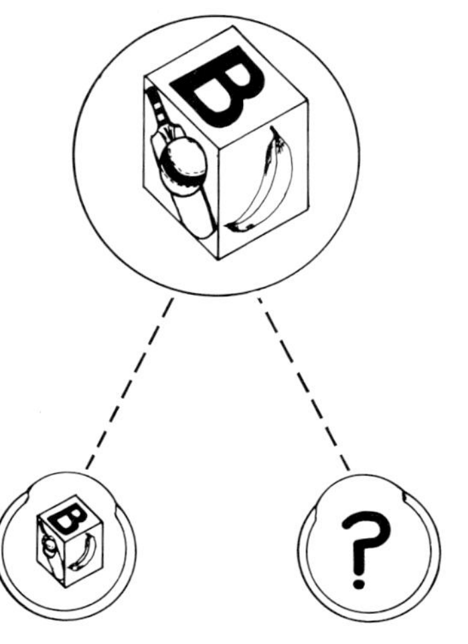


Amblyopia—sometimes referred to as lazy eye—is most commonly associated with a squint, but it need not be. An amblyopic eye shows a defect of acuity even though it seems to be structurally normal or has been provided with a spectacle lens suitable for compensating for any refractive anomaly. The cause of the condition is ill understood, but one element is disuse of the eye or misuse during the early years of life. Amblyopia in its true sense cannot arise in adults, though it can be used to describe a visual defect that occurs in an eye without any obvious structural changes. Most commonly this is due to the use of strong tobacco or drugs.

The photograph of a squint is reproduced by permission of the Institute of Ophthalmology; the photograph of epicanthus is reproduced from Miller, S J H, *Parson's Diseases of the Eye*, 16th edn, chapter 31, by kind permission of the publishers, Churchill Livingstone.

# REFRACTIVE ANOMALIES

## Disorders of shape and size

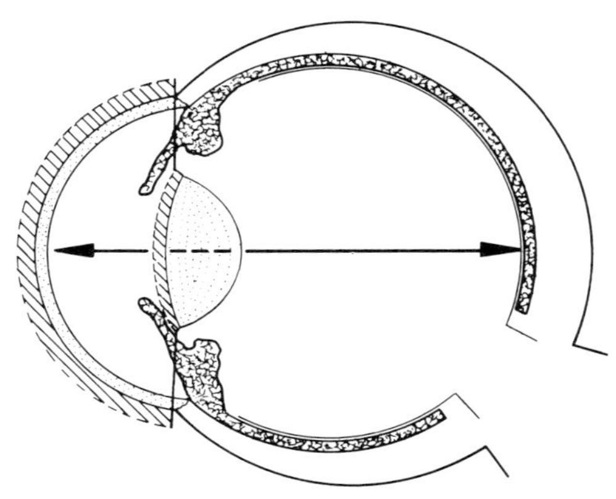

Refractive disorders are basically purely disorders of shape and size determined by inheritance and growth. Correct refraction depends on the distance between the cornea and the retina and its relation with the curvatures of both the cornea and the lens.

The three common disorders of refraction are hypermetropia (long sight), myopia (short sight), and astigmatism—which may exist on its own or in combination with either myopia or hypermetropia.

The long-sighted eye is too short from back to front, so that focused images cannot be focused on the retina but fall behind it. Conversely, the short-sighted eye is too long, and focused images from any distance may fall in front of the retina.

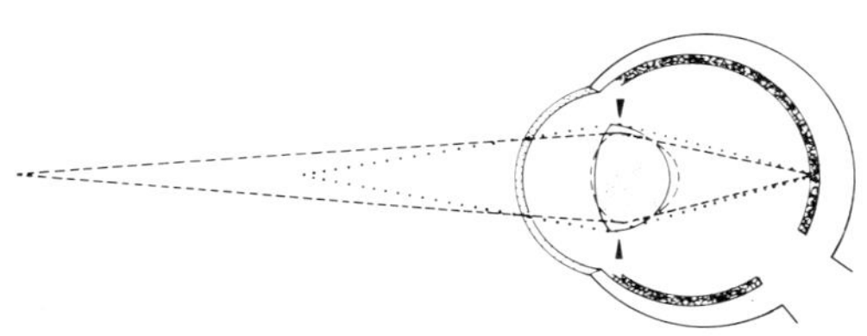

In any eye as an object comes closer its focused image within the eye moves further back. In short-sighted people there comes a point where it coincides with the retina: hence their ability to read without glasses, though they may be severely handicapped for distance vision.

The defect in hypermetropia is slightly different. Although the nearer an object comes to the eye the further backwards the image is focused, this backward movement may be completely or only partially neutralised by accommodation. Accommodation plays no essential part in myopia.

## Accommodation: changing the curvature of the lens

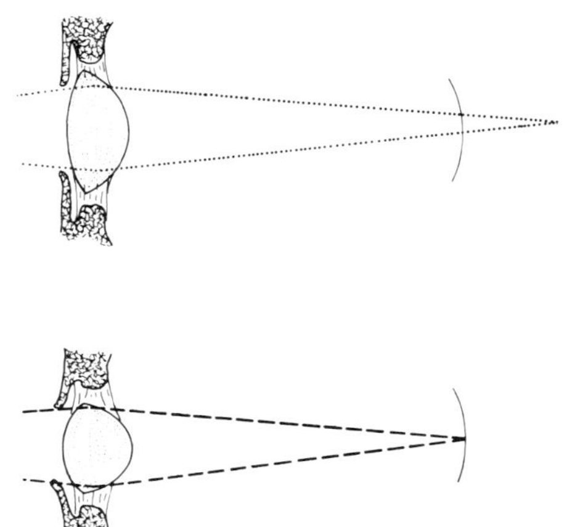

Curvature of the lens is the only dimension in the eye over which there is commonly any control. Normally the eye is "set" for distance, but the lens can be squeezed by its controlling muscle (the ciliary muscle) to give greater magnification and accurate focusing for near work such as reading. This is known as accommodation. When the pressure is released the lens, being elastic, resumes its normal shape. The amount of adjustment that can be obtained through accommodation is limited, so small near objects for many people are impossible. The ability to accommodate is greatest in children and progressively diminishes. This loss of accommodating ability produces difficulties with reading in the early 40s and is complete by the early 60s. This is because the lens gradually loses its elasticity and hardens and explains why people with previously normal vision need reading glasses in middle age.

# Refractive anomalies

## Astigmatism

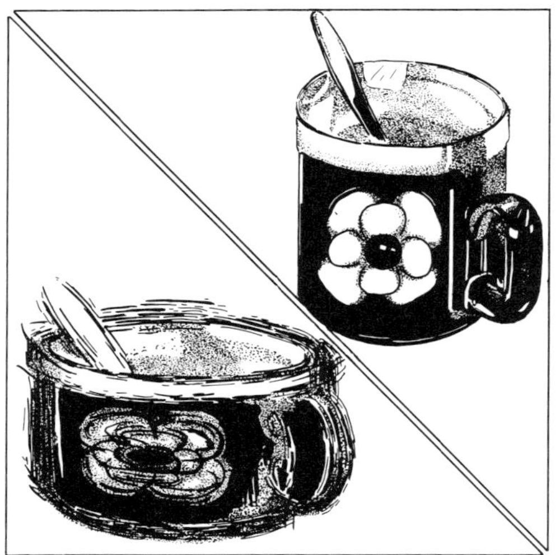

To produce a clear image the surface of a lens must be evenly curved. In astigmatism the curvature of the cornea differs according to whether it is measured horizontally or vertically. An image reaching the retina is therefore focused differently in one axis from the other. The effect is rather like the image in a distorting mirror.

Astigmatism may be superimposed on short- or long-sighted eyes, or it may be the only optical defect.

## Development in children

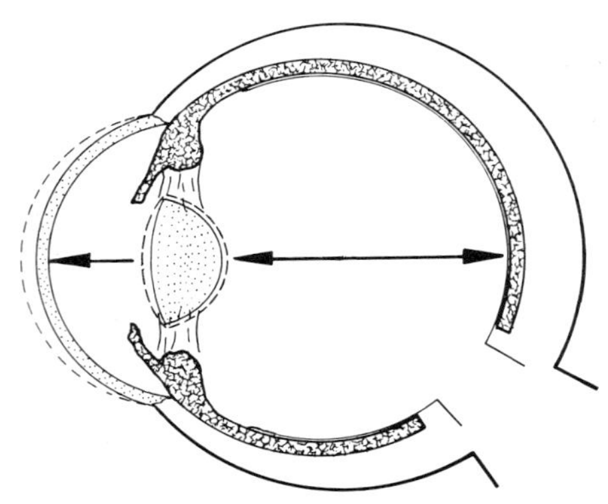


Normally changes in the curvature of the cornea and lens compensate for the effect of the increasing length of the eyeball that occurs during a child's growth. The notable exception is myopia. Children or adolescents who develop myopia not only have an eyeball longer than average but changes in the curvature of their cornea or lens are not adequate to compensate. Children rarely become myopic before the age of 6 (though a few are born myopic). The number of new cases increases from then on, reaching a peak at about 11.

The myopia usually gets intermittently worse until the late teens, when changes stop in most patients. This change is irreversible, and it is frequent enough in some children to warrant a change of glasses every six months. The unpredictability of the rate of change necessitates a review every six months or so.

Myopia seems to differ from hypermetropia in two respects. The changes in refraction during childhood and adolescence tend to be much greater in myopia than in hypermetropia, and a small percentage of myopic adults develop secondary degeneration of the retina and the vitreous, leading to a range of visual handicap in later life. These changes warrant an attitude of wariness towards myopia.

We do not know any way of preventing myopia, its progress, or its complications. The myopic child tends to be an achiever and should be given every encouragement to fulfil his potential.

## Dealing with defects in refraction

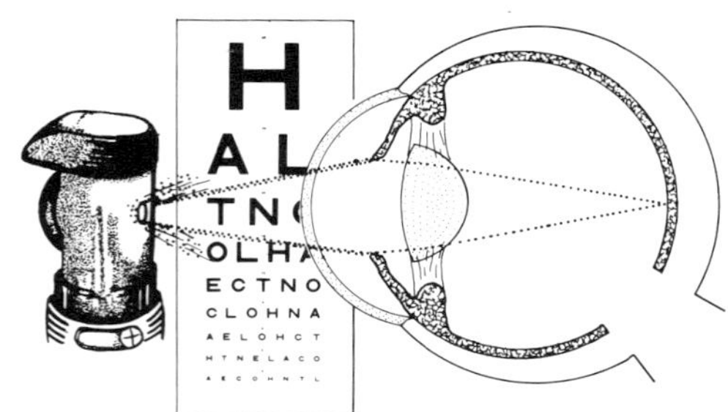

For any anomaly of refraction the decision whether to prescribe glasses must be based on the individual's visual difficulties, not on the refraction alone. In adults the use or disuse of glasses for long sight or short sight has no long-term effect on changes in vision. But young children with marked refractive anomalies should wear glasses or they may never reach their full visual potential.

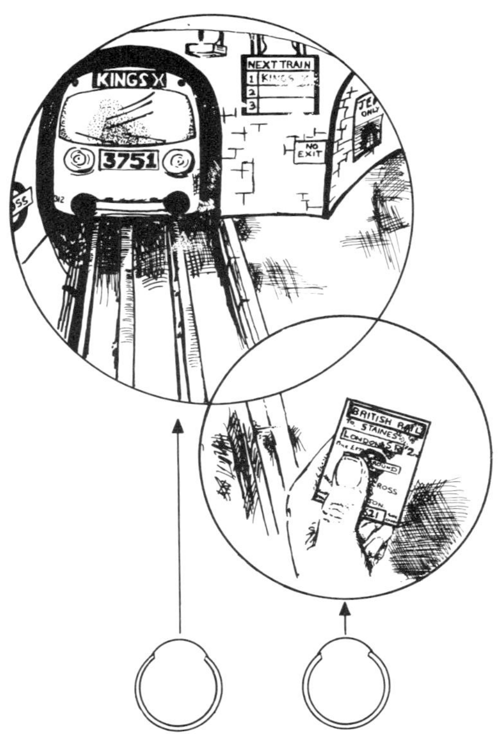

These optical abnormalities may be assessed by measuring the "refraction." The examiner flashes a light through varying lenses through the pupil to the back of the eye until an abnormality is neutralised. Theoretically this gives an absolute measurement of the abnormality and an accurate guide to the best prescription. But it does require some co-operation from the patient, so that children or confused people present difficulties.

The decision on the best glasses is not just a scientific one based on optical measurements but also a professional one based on an assessment of the person's need to see and how much he can tolerate. For example, some ophthalmologists use the bottom line on an eye chart as an example of intolerable visual detail for some people.

Since the presence of an optical defect is not a compelling criterion for prescribing compensating glasses, a middle-aged person who is slightly hypermetropic in one eye and slightly myopic in the other—that is, has optically imperfect eyes—can reasonably use his long-sighted eye for excellent distance vision and his short-sighted eye for minute reading vision. There are many other examples where glasses are unnecessary.

From this point of view, adults could well choose their own spectacles from a self-service store, but many serious visual disorders would be missed. For example, increasing myopia often occurs in people with incipient cataracts—changes in visual acuity should therefore always be investigated by specialists.

# Common misconceptions

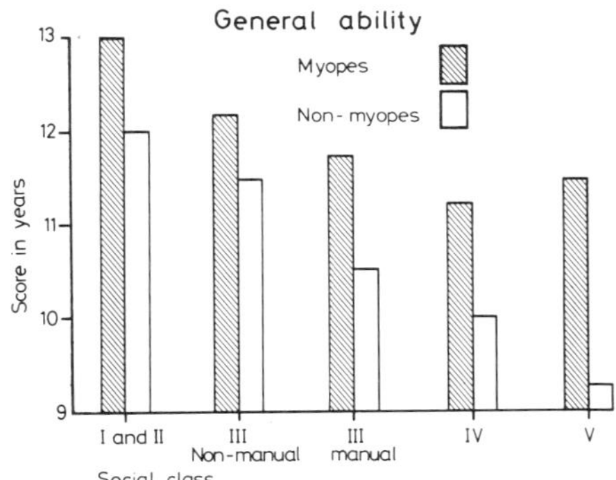


There is no known explanation for the breakdown in co-ordination of the growth of the eye that occurs in children with myopia, but there are several misconceptions. The commonest is that myopia is due to too much reading. There is no statistical evidence for this but it gains credibility because of the age at which myopia appears (that is, during school) and because of the correlation between myopia, social class, and academic achievement.

Both in the case of acquired myopia in children and in the other common acquired visual defect—presbyopia in middle age—people are inclined to confuse the fact that their vision tends to continue to deteriorate even after they have got spectacles with the thought that the spectacles cause the deterioration. Intrinsic changes in sight are not influenced by glasses at all, but in young children full visual potential may never be reached if glasses are not worn.

Another common fallacy is that eyestrain damages the eye. Use of the eye, even "excessive" use to the point of fatigue does not damage the eye, just as excessive physical exercise to the point of fatigue does not damage the legs. The brain, which has the job of interpreting the images, tires long before the eye can be harmed.

There is no proof that contact lenses have any effect on the changes that occur in myopia or any other refractive disorder. Because of their position on the eye a larger change in the basic myopia has to take place than with glasses before a visual loss is noticed.

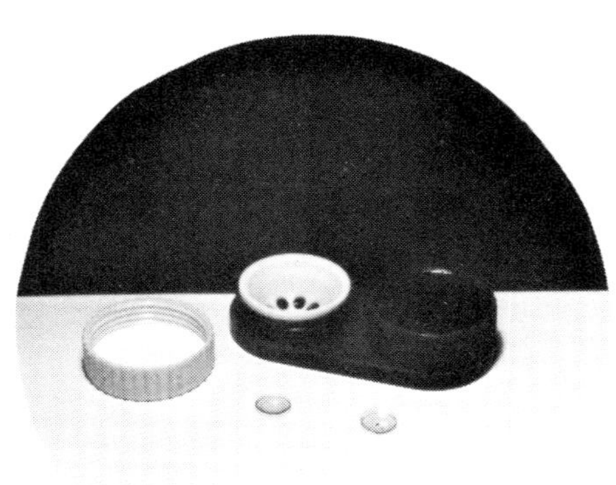

In conditions such as conical cornea, other corneal dystrophies, and unilateral aphakia contact lenses are extremely valuable. Tolerance and length of wear achieved by different people vary greatly and are usually unpredictable at the outset. Injuries resulting from faulty manipulation can be painful and even disabling. To some extent these complications can be lessened by using the soft variety, but these do not give such good vision. They also demand stringent hygiene and introduce the danger of infection. People working in dusty, windy atmospheres or where smoke or fumes occur are not likely to find contact lenses comfortable. Similarly, those with hay fever or other allergies may have special difficulties.

# METHODS OF EXAMINATION

## Sight testing

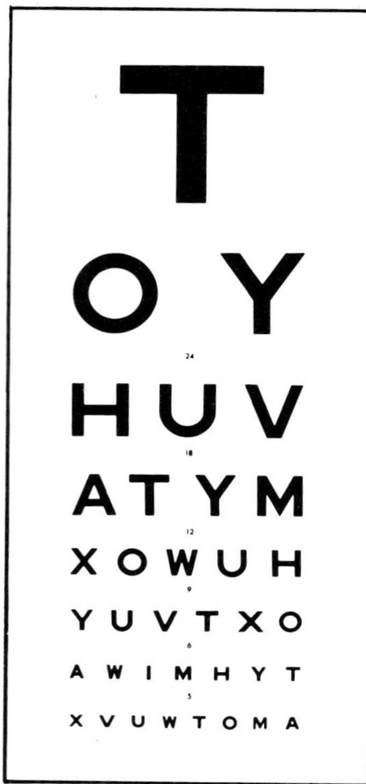

Though changes in eyesight are remediable by glasses more often than not, they may herald a change that has nothing to do with refraction but may instead be a precursor of serious handicap. Recording is therefore important.

The sight testing chart should be looked at from 6 metres (20 feet), or from 3 metres if looked at through a mirror. The last complete line that the patient can read completely accurately indicates his acuity in that eye.

Failure to read the top line should only be recorded when the patient has been brought closer to the chart until he can see. His vision may then be recorded as, for example, 4/60 or even less than 6/60. This is still useful vision without glasses, especially if near vision is normal.

Near vision is tested with print of standard type sizes at 25 cm or the distance the patient prefers. Normal vision is N5.

People who cannot read or cannot read Western script may be tested with a matching test, such as the Sheridan-Gardiner. The patient matches with his finger on a card the letter being shown. This test also has the advantage of being portable and so can be used for bedridden patients.

Whatever an eye looks like it is worse off if the visual acuity is affected than if it is not. An eye with symptoms that looks healthy and has good visual acuity should not be dismissed as necessarily normal, but its needs are less urgent than those of an eye with affected acuity.

The patient's own remarks about his sight are about as valuable as any he might make about his pulse. Sight tests should normally be carried out with glasses as the aim is to find out the best the eye is capable of.

## Testing colour vision

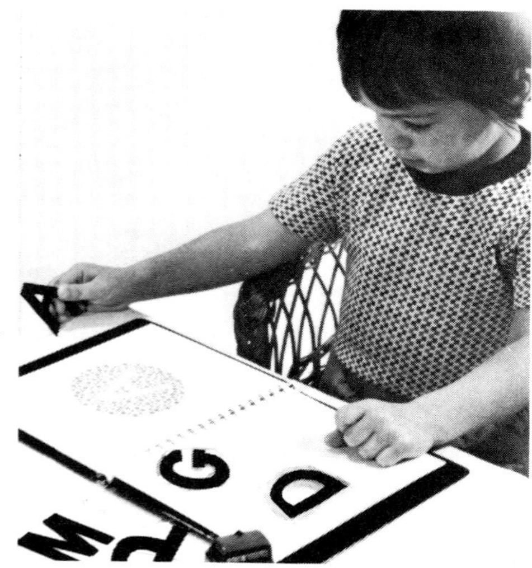

In rare cases (such as occurs, for example, in multiple sclerosis) acquired defects of colour vision may be diagnostically valuable, though they are usually overshadowed by other visual loss. Because the eye focuses red and blue light differently on the retina, even a minor defect of refraction can produce a variation in colour appreciation which disappears with correct glasses. Any disease, such as diabetes or glaucoma, which affects the cone cells of the retina may change colour values.

True colour blindness is so rare as to be unimportant for the average doctor. Defects in colour vision are, however, more common. Among Europeans about 8 in 100 boys and about 1 in 1000 girls inherit some difficulty in colour appreciation. It is usually well compensated for except in trick conditions. It is useful to expose these defects early, so that children and their teachers may foresee some difficulties. Useful tests are the Ishihara for adults and the Guy's colour vision test for children.

# Comparing two eyes for vision and appearance

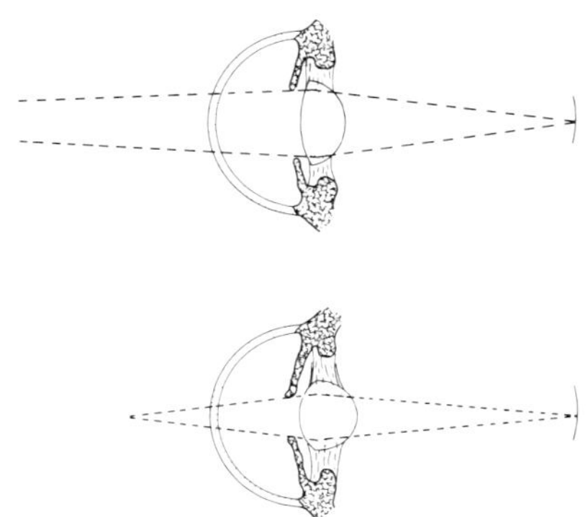


Equal performance of each eye with glasses for both near and distant vision is normal; unequal vision needs to be accounted for. Comparing one eye with the other is useful not only for acuity but also for: the size of the eye, separation of the lids, colour of conjunctiva and iris, size, shape, and activity of the pupils, and brightness of the cornea.

Most discrepancies can be detected in good light without any instruments, though a torch and magnifying lens are useful.

# Pupils: size and speed of reaction

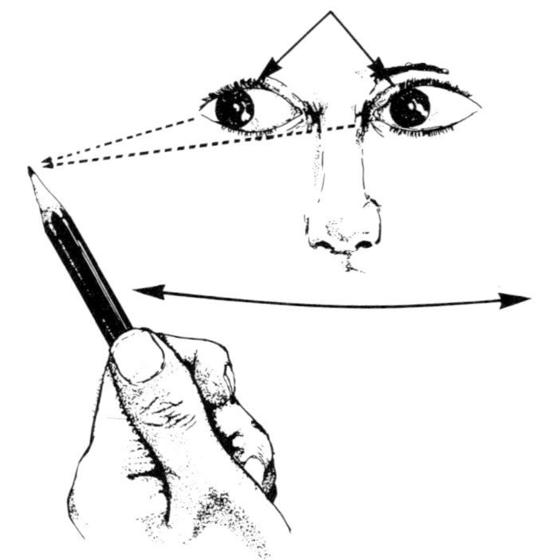

Pupil reactions are commonly missed because differences are often very small, both in size and speed of reaction. Most reactions are exaggerated in the dark so conclusive evidence may be obtained only in a dark room test. The pupil constricts not only in response to light, but also to focus for near vision. Failure to constrict to either light or near vision is an important sign. Any difference between the pupils in size or reaction needs explaining. In the absence of any neurological symptoms the wisest course is to refer to an ophthalmologist.

# Eye movements

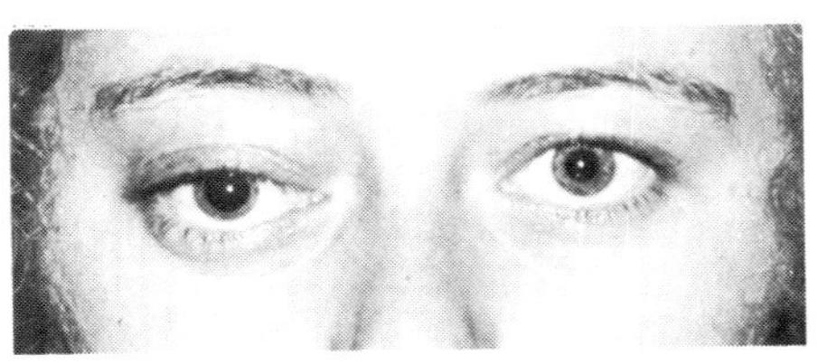

Eye movements may be tested by asking the patient to follow an object held in the hand, such as a pencil point. Movements should be equally full in both eyes in all directions, though the many people who suffered a squint in childhood might have these movements somewhat modified. The importance of this is minimal in adults unless there are new visual symptoms, the likeliest being double vision.

In testing eye movements the patient should not be asked to perform the impossible feat of looking beyond the normal range of vision: he will produce intermittent fixation of the object, which it is easy to confuse with nystagmus.

# Lids

The lids too must be examined. The upper lids in particular must be symmetrical—this can be assessed by comparing the level at which they intersect the cornea. It is sometimes hard to decide whether the lower of the two or the higher is abnormal. Family photographs will help to show whether the difference in aperture is long standing. Normally, not only should the lid level be symmetrical; when the eyes are raised the lids should also move upwards symmetrically. A weakness of one or the other might indicate one of several neurological disorders, the most often missed being myasthenia gravis.

# Symmetry: determining the abnormal eye

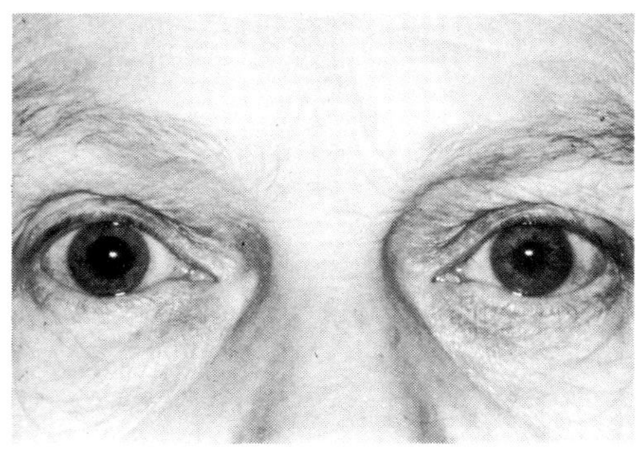

Symmetry of the two eyes depends not only on the equal function of the upper lid but also on the prominence of the globe. It is often difficult to determine which is the abnormal eye.

A small eye accompanied by a small pupil is a well recognised abnormality (Homer's syndrome), requiring investigation. Any eye that is becoming more prominent demands the exclusion of thyroid disease before considering disorders in the orbit that may be causing protrusion or deviation.

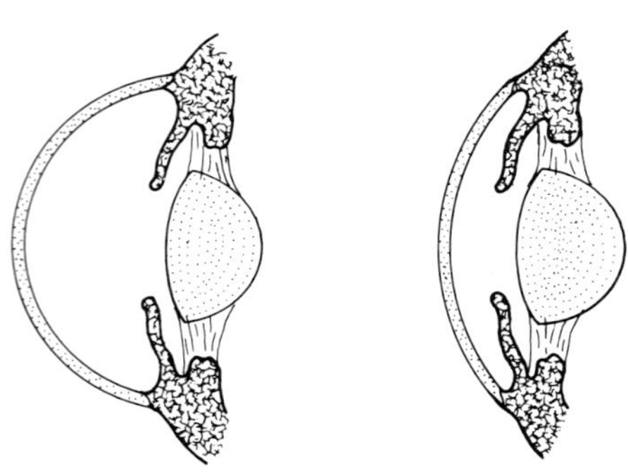

The distance in depth between the centre of the cornea and the plane of the iris should be identical in each eye. It is a serious sign if it is less in one eye than in the other, raising the possibility of glaucoma or a predisposition to glaucoma.

A shallow anterior chamber on both sides is difficult to assess because there is no standard of comparison, but when it is extremely pronounced the possibility of glaucoma needs careful consideration. The anterior chamber tends to become shallower from youth to age. Women also tend to have a deeper anterior chamber than men, so extreme shallowness tends to be a more important feature in women.

# Examining the inner eye

No reliable information about the eye behind the iris can be gained without an ophthalmoscope, except in people with well-advanced cataracts, when the pupil will be grey or white.

The ophthalmoscope consists of a series of lenses graded so that all the different planes of the eye can be examined from front to back. Too often it is regarded merely as an instrument for looking at the retina. Routine examination should begin using the high + lenses and end with the lens (theoretically 0, but seldom so in practice) that brings the retina into focus. If this routine is not followed opacities in the lens and vitreous may be missed.

Since the long-sighted eye is a small eye and the myopic a large one, the retina is focused sooner in a long-sighted eye. Also more of the retina of a long-sighted eye can be seen without moving the ophthalmoscope than that of a myopic eye. Any degree of astigmatism will prevent accurate focusing of the retina and optic nerve, and possibly lead to a false diagnosis since blurring of the nerve head is a sign of its being swollen. All these effects can be neutralised by viewing the interior of the eye through the patient's glasses. Dilating the pupil with Mydrilate 0·5% (cyclopentolate) with or without phenylephrine 10% helps to reduce any light reflections and increases the field. Immediately after examination the dilating drops should be neutralised with a constricting agent such as pilocarpine 2% or eserine (physostigmine) 0·25%. Known glaucomatous eyes should be left to the expert, as dilatation could be risky.

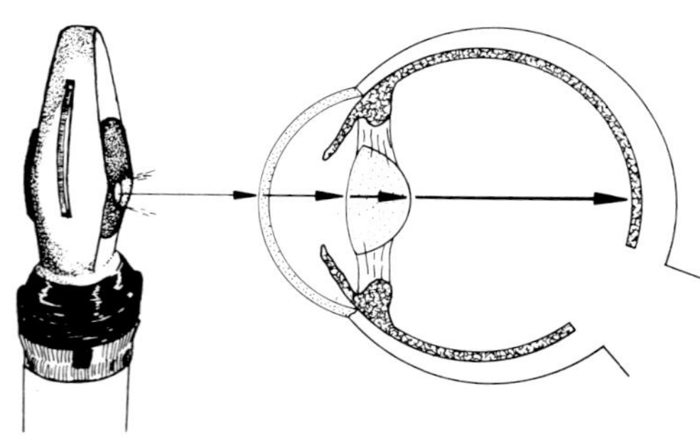


The examiner should stand alongside the patient and be as close to the patient's eye as possible. The examiner uses his right eye to examine the patient's right eye and his left to examine the patient's left. The patient should be asked to pretend to fix on a suitable object across the room.

# Through the eye

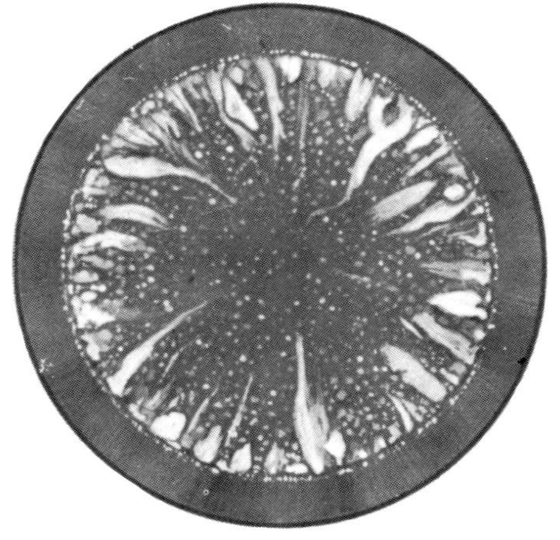

In a normal eye there is generally a featureless red glow until the retina is reached. Opacities in the cornea or lens show up as dark streaks or spots when the ophthalmoscope is focused at the appropriate depth and may be dense enough to prevent any view of the retina. Alternatively, some cataracts appear as a general haze or cloudiness.

The vitreous is normally completely transparent but it is relatively common for black threads or floating opacities of all shapes to be seen. To the patient these appear as floating marks when he views a light surface.

Any difficulty in seeing a clear picture of the retina may indicate serious intraocular disease and needs full investigation.

If there is no red reflex and a black pupil the probable cause is severe intraocular haemorrhage. Apart from trauma the commonest causes of haemorrhage are diabetes, arteriosclerosis, or hypertension.

# Retinal haemorrhage: a threat to vision

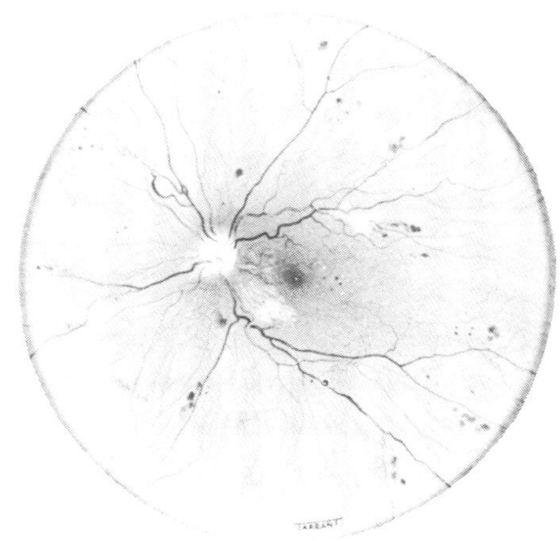

Any retinal haemorrhages are not only important because they are a threat to vision but also because they may indicate systemic disease such as hypertension, diabetes, anaemia, renal diseases, etc. Again a comparison between one retina and the other is often useful, and it is therefore good practice to dilate both pupils, even if the patient has symptoms in only one eye. The differential diagnosis of retinal abnormalities is difficult but any unusual picture needs investigation. Retinal haemorrhages vary in shape and size according to their cause, the vessel from which bleeding occurs, and the layer of the retina they are positioned in. They range from the pinpoint haemorrhage seen in some diabetics to the obvious chaotic patterns produced by thrombosis. All are potentially dangerous to life or sight and need an ophthalmological assessment as well as medical investigation.

As haemorrhages absorb they often leave white patches resembling exudate. Leakage of serum from the vascular bed also produces fluffy or discrete white areas dotted throughout the retina or in only one area. Where these are newly observed they require investigation just as much as haemorrhages, as they often indicate systemic disease. None of these necessarily produce easily detectable visual loss reported by the patient.

# Optic nerve heads: precise boundaries and central cup

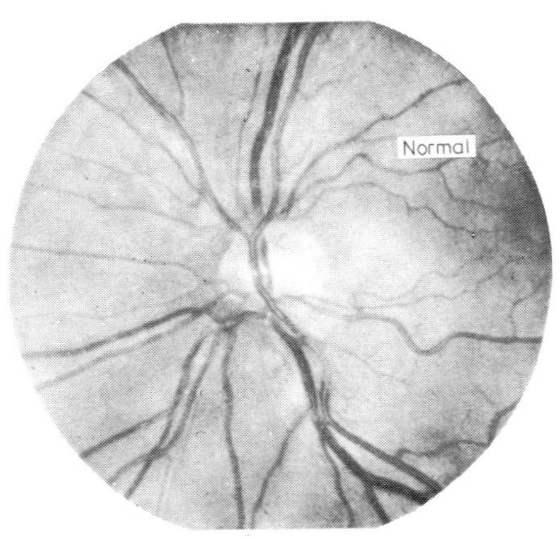


The optic nerve heads should have precise boundaries; neither should be paler than the other; and each should have a definite central cup. If the cup is not visible and the edges of the disc are blurred expert opinion is needed to exclude swelling caused by serious retro-ocular conditions.

A newly observed difference in pallor between the two eyes is more certainly an indication of the early stages of serious disease, especially in the absence of any history that may account for the difference. Equal pallor in both eyes is hard to evaluate, but if it is at all pronounced then further investigation is needed. Neurological signs elsewhere may be found, and even a small visual loss either of field or of acuity should be searched for.

# Methods of examination

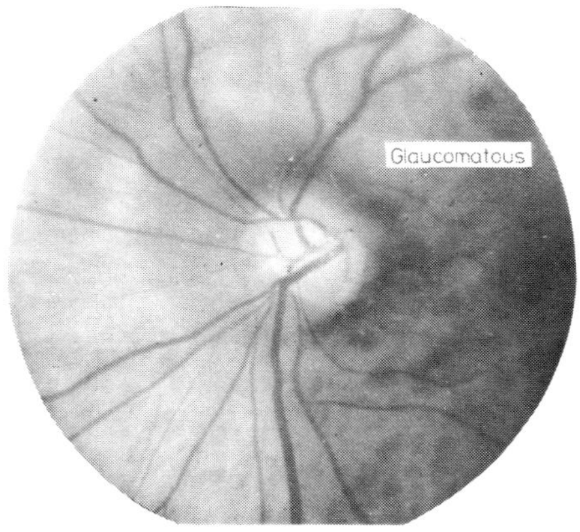



The normal cup has sloping sides and rounded edges. By contrast, a glaucomatous cup has sharp edges; in advanced cases the side of the cup extends behind the plane of the edge, so that the edge hides the blood vessels as they loop over and reappear further down in the nerve head. Hence in glaucoma a portion of the vessels cannot be seen, whereas in normal discs there is no such break in visibility as the vessels traverse the nerve head. Whatever the state of visual acuity, cupping of this nature, even in only one segment of the disc, warrants full scale investigation for glaucoma.

Swelling of the nerve head, featured by blurring of the disc margin, may indicate a serious disorder of cardiovascular or intracranial origin.

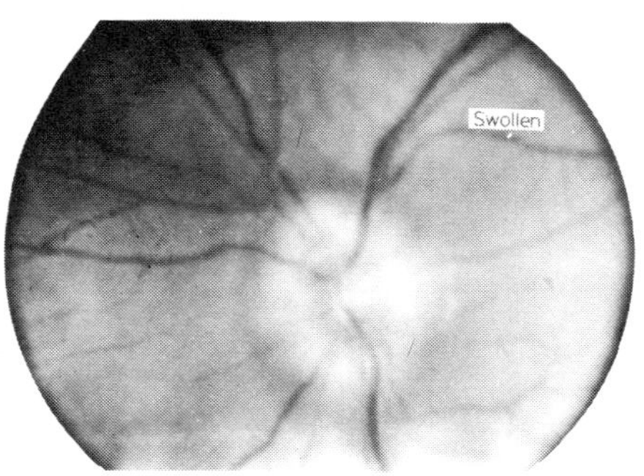



The position of retinal lesions is described by taking the optic nerve as the centre of a clock and measuring the distance from the disc as disc diameters. Thus a lesion may be 2 disc diameters from the disc at 3 o'clock. The closer a lesion is to the posterior pole of the eye the greater the immediate effect on vision may be. Even minute disturbances around the macula can affect near vision only, mainly because of the great concentration here of cone receptors, which are responsible for transmitting detailed impulses through the optic nerve.

Ophthalmoscopic investigation can be supplemented in cases where there is no visible lesion but some visual defect by dye injections and electrical tests.

The blood supply to this area often fails in old age. This accounts for the inability of some old people to read, though their distance vision is less severely affected. Close examination of the macula in these cases will often show abnormal fine or coarse pigment stippling. The visual handicap is often out of all proportion to the minute changes seen in the retina.

# Visual fields: central defects affect acuity

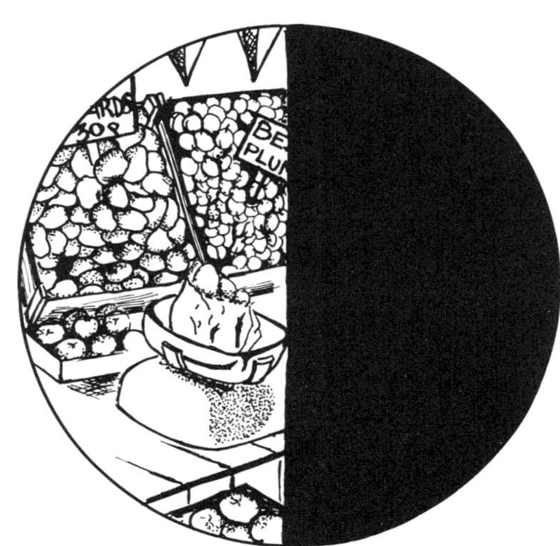



No examination of the eye is complete without assessing the visual fields. Some quite puzzling visual complaints become explicable when field defects are discovered. Most elderly people who have half their visual field obliterated (hemianopia) do not complain of this: they may mention only difficulty in reading or in mobility because of bumping into objects.

Unfortunately, testing the visual fields is not easy and in children up to the age of 10 even with instruments is often not more than a probable estimate. The minute telescopic central field of the glaucomatous is often described by a sufferer as "difficulty in getting about." Gross defects may be detected simply by the examiner stretching out his arms and asking the patient to fix on his nose. The examiner then moves the fingers of his hands. Any inaccuracy in the patient's response to these movements indicates some field loss in the temporal fields. If the patient then closes one eye any field defects in the nasal field of the other eye can be determined by comparison either with the examiner's own or with the fellow eye. The upper and lower fields can be investigated in a similar way. Disturbance of the central field is usually accompanied by some loss of acuity. This does not occur when the peripheral field is contracted.

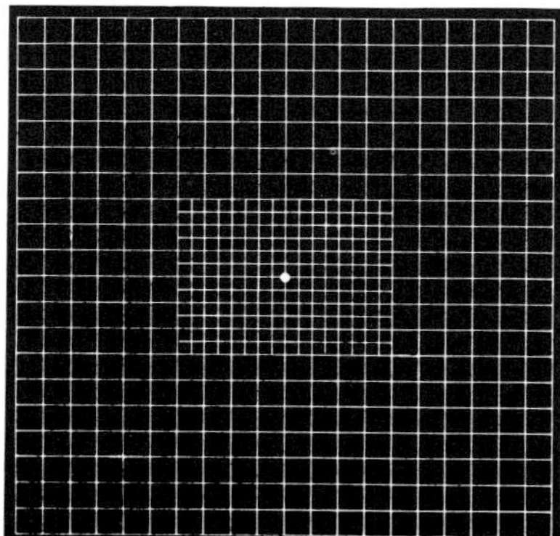

There are many types of field defect, but the finer ones have to be detected by instruments. Nevertheless, the results are still largely determined by the patient's subjective responses and these are often inaccurate. Possibly the most useful aid in the consulting room is the small book of Amsler charts. These enable small but diagnostic defects of the central field to be detected quickly and often accurately.

The photograph of the colour vision test is reproduced by permission of Keeler Instruments Ltd; those of asymmetrical eyelids, Horner's syndrome, lens opacities, retinal haemorrhage, and optic discs by permission of the Institute of Ophthalmology.

# GLAUCOMA

## A common disease

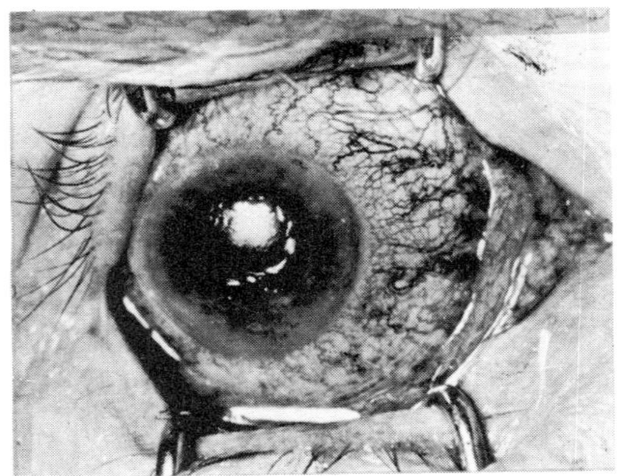

In the UK about 1% of people aged over 40 years and about 5% of those over 65 develop glaucoma; the proportion rises even higher among those of 80 or more. There is little difference between the sexes. Though there are congenital and juvenile forms, these are extremely rare outside families with known victims. After the age of 40 glaucoma should feature seriously in the list of possible diagnoses of eye disease.

## A blinding disease

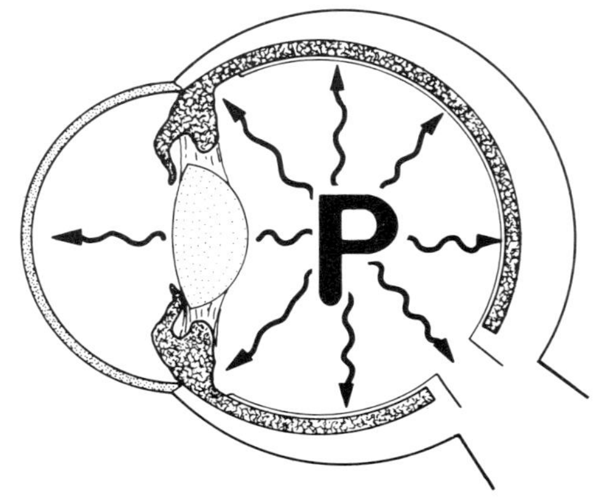


If left untreated glaucoma is a blinding disease, and early diagnosis and treatment are therefore crucial. Treatment can control the disease and limit visual loss, and the earlier it is started the more vision will be preserved.

The intraocular pressure is usually higher than normal in glaucoma, though the relation between the increase in pressure and its effect on visual function is uncertain. Some eyes tolerate a high pressure, while others do not: there is a condition called low-tension glaucoma. The range of normal values is wide (16-22 mm Hg) with diurnal variations of 3-5 mm Hg. Figures of tension are therefore unreliable as absolute diagnostic or prognostic weapons even when measured by tonometry. Digital methods tend to be inaccurate even in practised hands.

## Loss of vision: quick or slow



The increased pressure interferes with the transparency of the cornea and with the function of the retina, blunting its conduction of impulses, ultimately to the point of extinction.

This loss of vision may occur suddenly over a few days. Or it may be such a slow process that it takes many years before any significant loss can be measured, and the patient may not be aware of the loss because the last function to go is visual acuity for detail.

# Glaucoma

## Clinical presentation varies

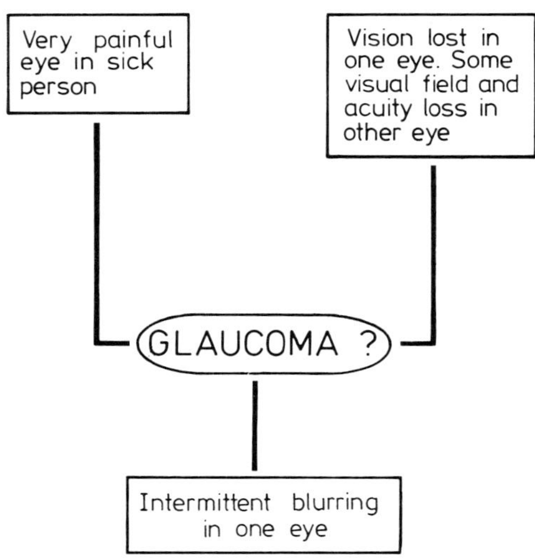


In ordinary clinical practice the problems are not those of measuring tension correctly but of being sure not to miss the signs that a sick person might be ill because of glaucoma. The condition varies considerably in presentation. The eye may be acutely painful and the patient very sick, or the eye may have been giving only mild intermittent trouble for weeks or months before the patient mentions it. Occasionally one eye may have failed completely and the other have lost much visual field or acuity before the patient seeks help.

Although the type of glaucoma—open angle or narrow angle—has a considerable effect on the type of treatment, in general practice it is rarely necessary to differentiate if an ophthalmologist's opinion is to be sought.

A patient aged over 40 who presents with headache, possibly very severe, may have acute or subacute glaucoma. The headache is often accompanied by nausea and vomiting. Indeed the abdominal symptoms may predominate. The fact that one eye is redder than the other or has severely reduced vision may not be reported or noticed. If it is noticed its presence may be thought to be mere coincidence. This may be a disastrous assumption: even an eye with previously normal sight may be irretrievably damaged in a few days if it is untreated. Alternatively the clinical episode might represent the final blow to an eye that had been quietly glaucomatous for some time.

## Blurring and rainbows

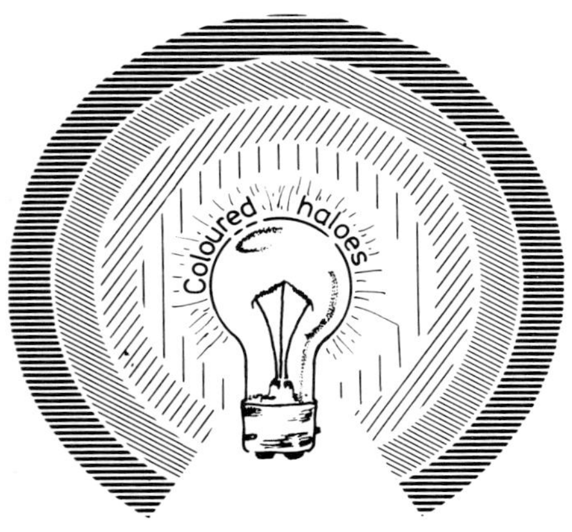


Although glaucoma can attack eyes that were previously normal there are two important early symptoms: blurring and rainbows round lights.

Blurring is intermittent but occurs at more or less regular intervals—sometimes at particular times of day. Attacks last from a few minutes to three-quarters of an hour and may be accompanied by headache, which is usually confined to the temporal area. The blurring, which may be only slight, affects both near and distant vision.

Patients should also be asked whether they see coloured haloes or rainbows around lights. Textbooks usually call this a halo, but a glaucomatous halo is invariably coloured. An unequivocal story of haloes around lights is evidence of glaucoma, irrespective of any other symptoms that might or might not be present.

## Pupils unequal and sluggish

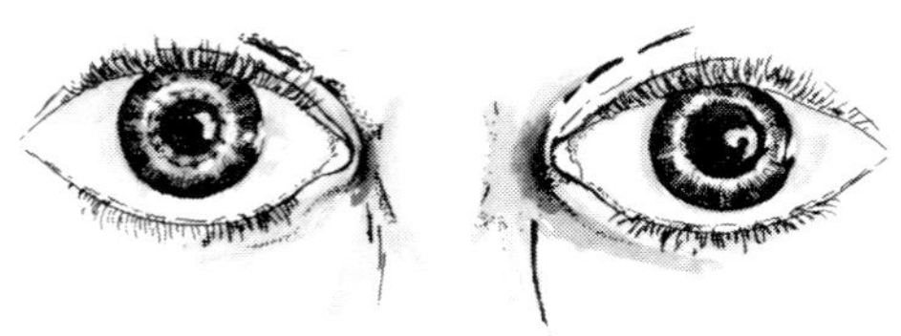

The state of the pupil is a valuable sign in the consulting room. Characteristically a glaucomatous pupil is either larger than its partner or more sluggish to light, or both. The difference in size may be very slight: only in the more acute or subacute glaucoma is the classical fixed dilated pupil found.

Both a large pupil and one that is sluggish need investigation on their own account, but they are reliable indicators of possible symptomless glaucoma. One difficulty lies in thinking that the smaller pupil is at fault. But this is not serious if pupil inequality is given its full weight and ophthalmological opinion sought. The chief difficulty lies in forgetting to look at the size of the pupils and their response to light.

Redness is common in acute glaucoma, but it is only a small part of the picture, which is dominated by pain, a dilated pupil and a clouded cornea. In chronic glaucoma the sclera and conjunctiva are normal in colour. Therefore neither the presence of redness nor its absence is a help.

# Well-defined optic discs: a late finding

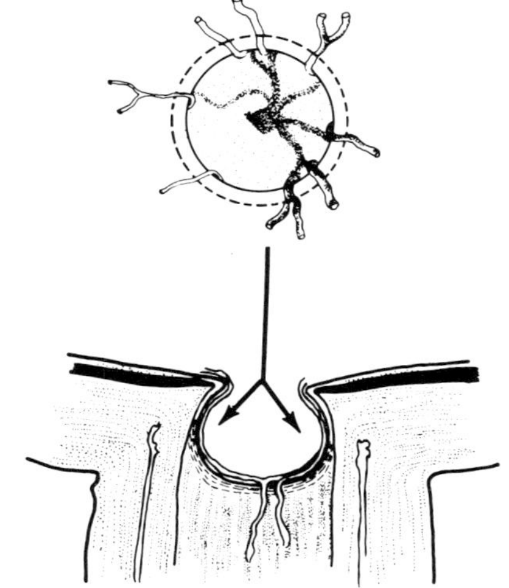

The glaucomatous disc is well defined when fully developed. In its early stages, however, it is no more than a very sharp edge, often in only one sector, and it needs considerable experience to recognise it.

By the time full cupping has appeared the disease is far advanced. Full cupping is therefore not a sign to wait for before seeking a diagnosis.

# Field defects and field loss

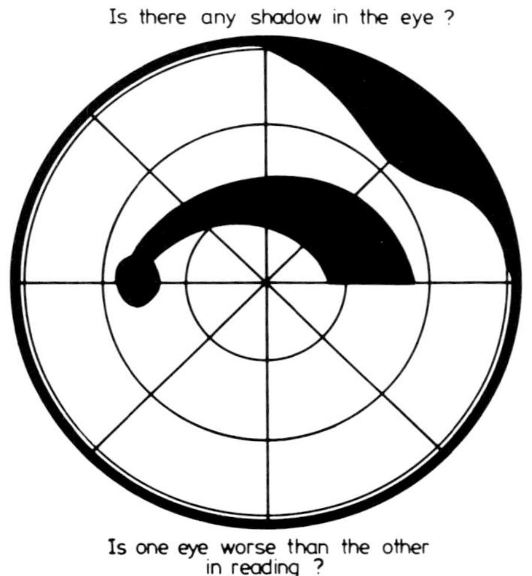


Field defects are hard to find in the early stages, except with special instruments. But the patient should be asked whether there appears to be a shadow in the eye and whether there is any difference in the ability to read very small print between one eye and the other with glasses. If this ability is tested many patients with glaucoma will produce evidence of a possible field defect.

The detection of field loss is the most important single measure in diagnosing glaucoma. At all stages of the disease the degree of field loss will show how seriously the disease is progressing and indeed whether it exists as any more than a potential threat to vision. The loss may be peripheral or central.

The most important loss is of any portion of the central field because this affects acuity. Central field loss may be an early sign. It may first express itself as letter missing in a line of small print, often described (if it is mentioned) merely as "difficulty with reading." The Amsler chart is particularly useful in elucidating central defects.

# When to suspect glaucoma

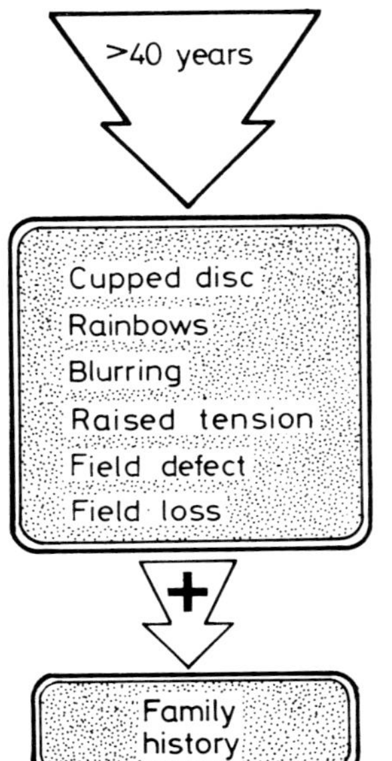


Any of these symptoms and signs should lead to the suspicion of glaucoma in anyone aged over 40, particularly if there is a family history of glaucoma.

Patients often do not know how to describe their relatives' eye conditions. But the fact that middle-aged or elderly relatives have visited hospital for their eyes and have used drops is evidence that they might have had glaucoma. If there is a family history extensive investigation is justified even if symptoms are only minor and confused.

Opinions differ about screening for glaucoma in people over 40 with a family history and about the frequency of observation in those suspected of having the condition. But people with suspicious symptoms (and their relatives) should be warned of the possible changes and told to look out for episodic blurring or coloured haloes.

# Glaucoma

## Management

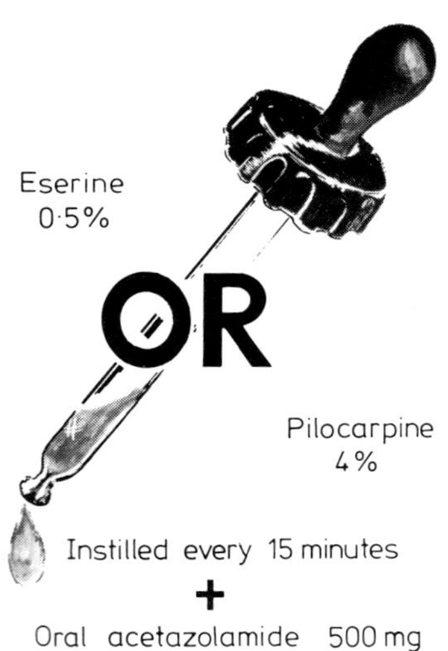



Management may be complex and protracted. Even so the GP can take simple measures to prevent unnecessary complications. Many patients have to use drops over many years to control the disease. Drops can be extremely effective, but their use must be uninterrupted. Two bottles of drops should always be issued at the same time. If only one is prescribed and then spilt patients tend to wait until their next visit to hospital before asking for more. Except immediately after operation, patients should not be deterred from using their only available drops by the fact that the time on the date stamp has expired: it is safer to use out-of-date drops than not to use any. They should also take their drops as usual when they are on holiday, and if they forget them they must seek help, however difficult this may be.

A GP who suspects glaucoma in a patient and finds it hard to arrange emergency admissions would be wise to instil a miotic. If there is no glaucoma this will do no harm, and if there is it may save sight and will confirm the diagnosis if the symptoms are greatly relieved.

The miotic (eserine 0·5% or pilocarpine 4%) should be instilled every 15 minutes for one hour into the eye with a dilated or sluggish pupil, and acetazolamide (500 mg) should also be given once by mouth. This procedure should be performed only in cases of acute glaucoma.

## Precipitating factors: 56 drugs

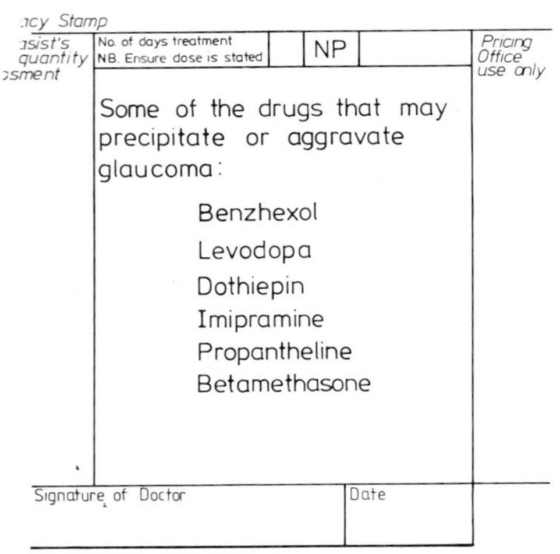



There are 56 drugs in common use that may precipitate glaucoma or aggravate it. The commonest are those that have an action similar to that of atropine—for example, many gastrointestinal drugs—and those given to control tremor or rigidity, as in Parkinson's disease. Any reports from patients about treatment are likely to be garbled, and even if accurate an optician might not recognise the implications. Likewise, few ophthalmologists can identify pills and capsules from a description of their shape and colour. As well as being aware of the effects of treatment on eye conditions, GPs are well placed to give relevant details to ophthalmologists.

There is also a psychosomatic element in glaucoma. The blurring of vision that may occur in people under stress may be wrongly attributed to the stress. The blurring might instead be due to the glaucoma and the treatment for stress might actually precipitate attacks of glaucoma.

## Conclusion

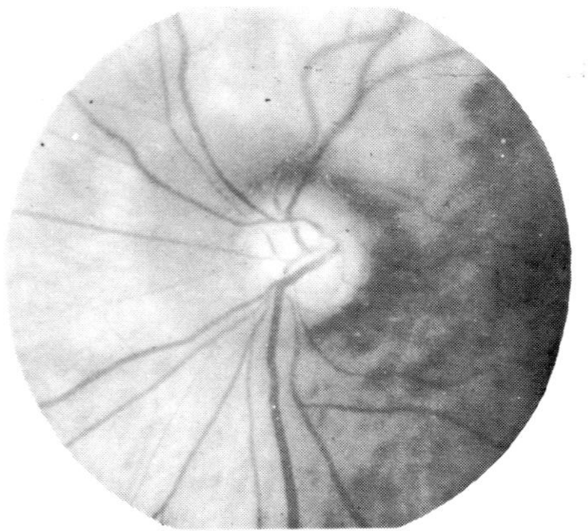

Glaucoma must be considered in any patient over 40 who has blurred vision. If the patient also sees coloured haloes round lights he almost certainly has glaucoma. The important signs are dilated and sluggish pupils.

The GP's difficulty is to know which patients he should refer to hospital for extensive investigation and which can rely on services outside hospital such as opticians and medical eye centres. Certainly all patients with typical symptoms should attend hospital. As with other ocular diseases, the threshold for referral must be much lower if the eye under suspicion is the better one.

The photograph of an eye suffering from acute glaucoma is reproduced from *An Atlas of Diseases of the Eye* by kind permission of Dr Peter Hansell and Churchill Livingstone Ltd; that of glaucomatous cupping is reproduced by permission of the Institute of Ophthalmology.

# CATARACTS

## Senile cataract: the commonest problem

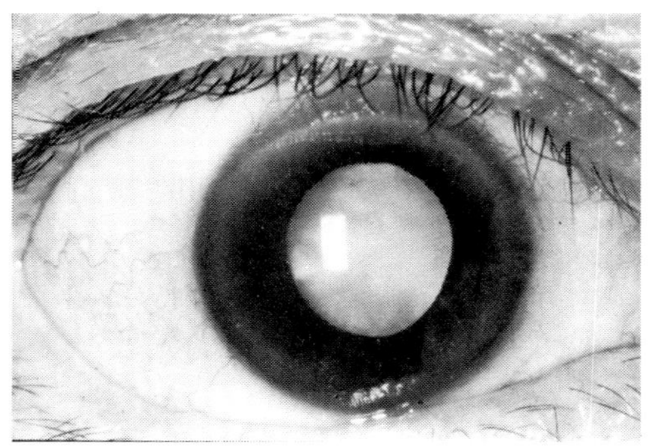

There are various types of cataract—congenital, juvenile, traumatic, toxic, and secondary. Far more common than all these put together, however, are senile cataracts.

The optical problems are broadly the same whatever the age of the patient, though management and assessment of cataracts in the elderly tend to be more straightforward.

## Lens opacities impair vision

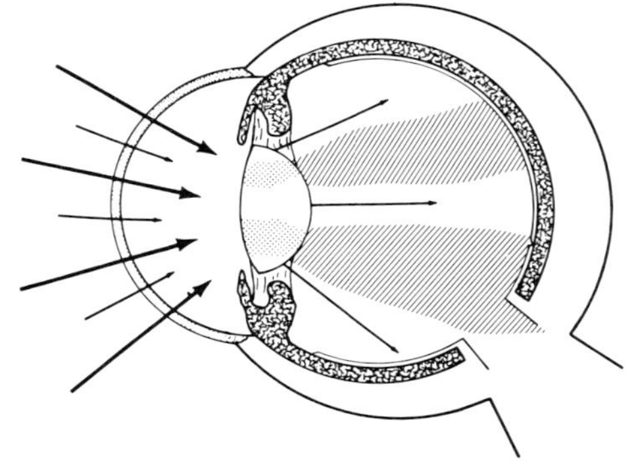

The retina depends for its stimulation on the transparency of all the structures in front of it—the vitreous, lens, cornea, and aqueous. In cataract, the lens loses its transparency, either overall or in spots or stripes that resemble the flaws in imperfect glass. Cataract is therefore internal and invisible without instruments until the lens becomes completely opaque. When it reaches this state it appears as a greyish-white pupil.

The common senile cataract, as opposed to a traumatic or inflammatory one, is always formed gradually. To the patient it seems as if he is looking through glass that is gradually frosting. Even when fully developed light can always be perceived, and shadowy movements can usually also be seen.

## Natural history of senile cataracts

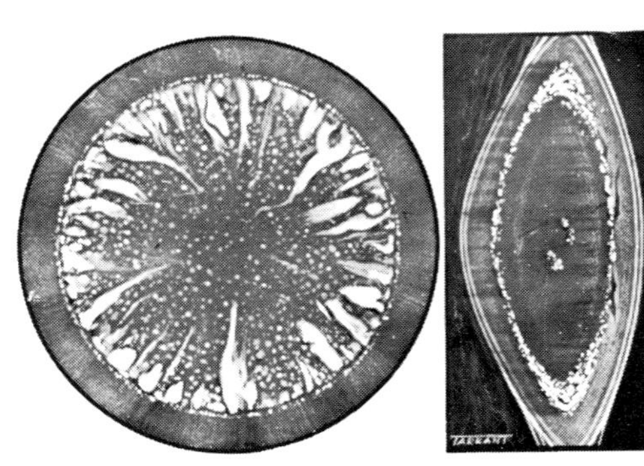

Senile cataract rarely occurs before the age of 55 in temperate climates in well-nourished healthy people. Given longevity mild opacification of the lens will almost inevitably occur, though not to the extent of becoming a handicap. As this is unlikely to impair a patient's activities it is best not described as a cataract.

In general, the younger the patient, the more rapidly cataract progresses, though vision often deteriorates in fits and starts. Indeed, progression is not inevitable, and nobody can forsee the rate at which opacities will increase, nor the extent to which they will develop. There is no medical treatment that will halt the decline or improve vision. Conversely, nothing will accelerate the progress.

One possible exception to this general rule is in patients with diabetes, in whom cataracts occur earlier and often progress more rapidly than normal. Observation needs to be no more frequent than once every six months, unless there are special features or obvious deterioration over a shorter period.

## Removing the lens: the only real treatment

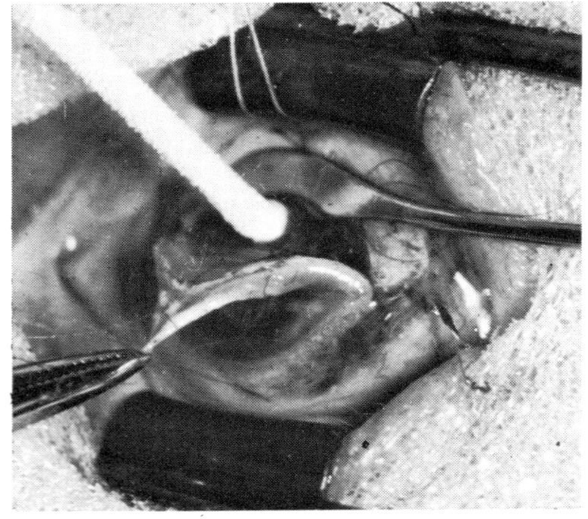

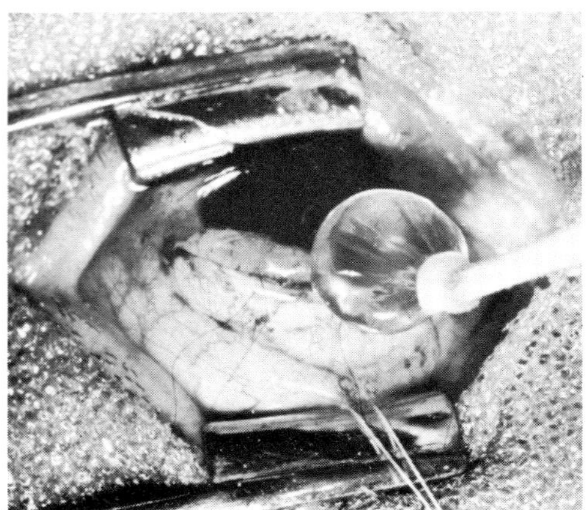

In the early stages of cataract formation the refractive changes that often occur can be compensated for by glasses. Surgery to remove the lens is, however, the only real treatment for cataract. Surgery can (and should) be performed in an otherwise healthy eye as soon as visual handicap is serious.

Patients' needs differ and surgeons' approaches vary, but in nearly everyone the lens can be extracted safely, whatever its state. The operation may be performed under local or general anaesthesia, and no more than a day or two of bedrest afterwards is needed. Most elderly patients can be assured of a technically successful outcome.

Only among the elderly confused does the operation tend to be unsuccessful. Surgery often exacerbates the confusion, even though the practice of padding the eyes after operation is no longer so common as it used to be.

When cataracts are present in both eyes double extractions are increasingly being considered, though both lenses are rarely removed on the same day. A double extraction means the patient's visual environment is totally changed.

Many people need re-education after cataract extraction anyway, and the lack of any previous visual reference after a double operation can be a burden. On the other hand, if the second operation is not done at the same time as the first some patients find it difficult to return to the theatre and prefer discharge. Much depends on the vision in the second eye and the temperament of patient and surgeon.

## Substitute lenses may cause problems

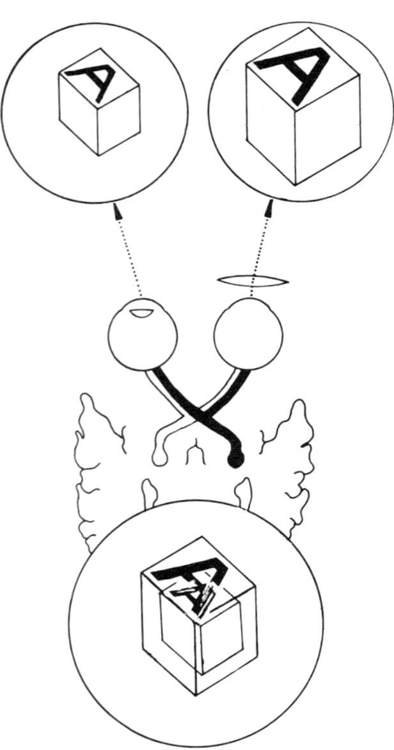

To see accurately again after the lens has been removed the eye needs a substitute lens. Ideally the replacement should go in the same position as the original lens. This is technically possible but has complications so the lens is usually provided as spectacles. Because of its position away from the eye the spectacle lens has to have more magnification than the natural one to provide an accurate focus.

If the patient's other eye still has adequate vision then it will transmit a normal-sized focused image. The brain will therefore be confronted with two clear images of the same object but of different sizes, which it cannot merge. A contact lens worn on the eye is near enough to the actual position of the natural lens to overcome this difficulty, but the elderly often cannot manipulate contact lenses.

When only one cataract is removed, the eye with the better vision being left, the operation is really done as an insurance against the better eye suddenly failing. Should it do so the other eye and its spectacle lens can immediately take over. Without this precaution the patient would be effectively blind till surgery could be performed.

# Magnification and distortion after removal

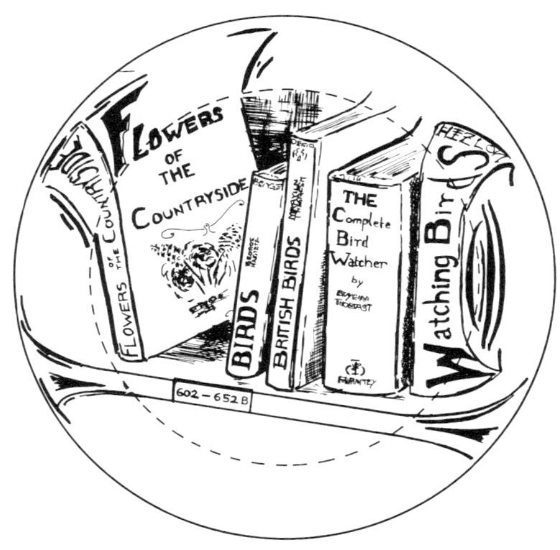



The magnification produced by correctly focused spectacles is also a trouble to many when both eyes rely on spectacle lenses. People who rely predominantly on size to give clues to distance have difficulty in judging distance because of the magnification of the image produced by their spectacle lenses.

Not only the magnification causes difficulty: only the centre of a powerful spectacle lens gives a focused image, and people who were formerly able to use their peripheral field confidently become confused by the lens's distortion.

Contact lenses provide the solution to both these problems, but glasses for reading and near work are needed to supplement the contact lenses because after removal of the lens the eye cannot accommodate. If the patient does not have contact lenses but relies on spectacles then he will need two pairs—for near and for far vision—or a pair of bifocals to overcome the loss of accommodation. Appreciable changes in refraction rarely occur later than three months after cataract extraction, so a change in acuity in the elderly any time after this is probably caused by some other condition irrelevant to glasses.

# The general practitioner's role

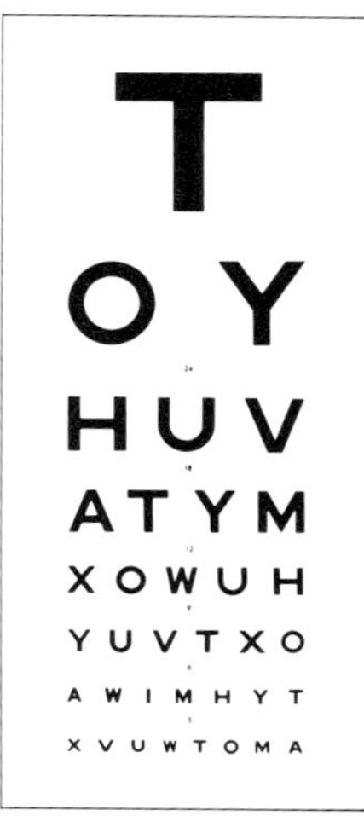



If the general practitioner is told by an optician that one of his patients has cataracts that seem to be progressing, he should follow this up by examining the patient when he next attends or by inviting him for examination. Then he can assess whether or not a hospital visit is necessary, taking account of the patient's personality and general health.

If the general practitioner measures the patient's acuity himself and it appears adequate, then repeat measurements will show clearly whether there is any deterioration and whether the patient needs referring. If patients are worried about their visual deterioration there is little problem, but they often cover up because of fear, or they may be unaware of the changes.

# Surgery useless if retina unhealthy

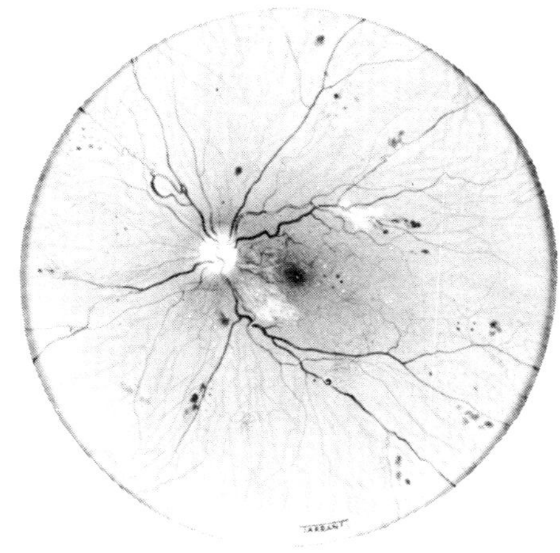

One of the major difficulties facing ophthalmologists who see elderly people with well developed cataracts for the first time is to know whether their retina is healthy. If the retina is degenerate or unhealthy for other reasons, such as diabetes, surgery will provide little or no benefit. This is a good reason for expert examination in the early stages of cataract formation and a reason for referral to a medical ophthalmologist.

Most ophthalmologists need to know about any other disease or disability the patient may be suffering from and any drugs he is taking. Patients will often deny having any constitutional disease, and about half the elderly patients who deny any illness forget that they are having preventive treatment of some sort.

The information that the general practitioner can provide on the patient's general health may therefore be an invaluable aid to diagnosis and to choosing the right form of treatment.

Photographs of mature cataract, lens opacities, removal of a lens, and retinopathy are reproduced by permission of the Institute of Ophthalmology.

# VISUAL DIFFICULTY IN OLD AGE

## Visual problems change with age

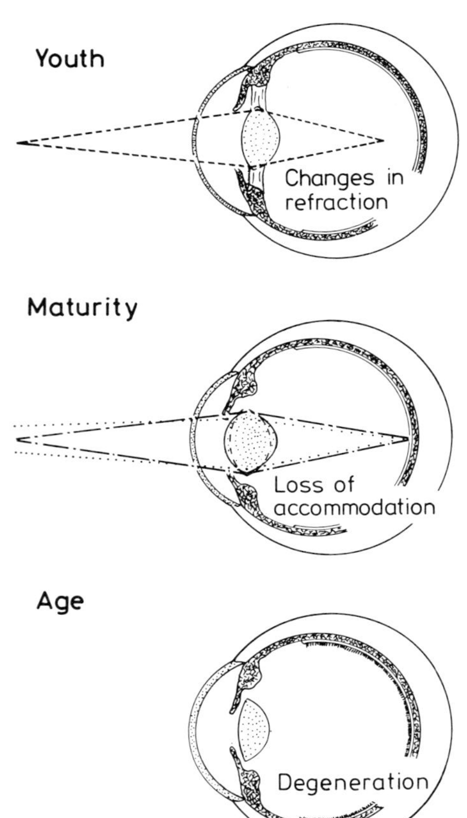



So far as vision is concerned, there are three periods of life: up to the age of 20 (development); from 20 to 60 (maturity); and after 60 (the old eye).

These ages are characterised by the changes in refraction that occur in some children and adolescents; changes in the power of accommodation and the difficulties of the hypermetrope that occur in the latter half of middle age; and the absence of any refractive change in old age except those secondary to disease and degeneration.

Before the age of 60 nearly all disorders of eyesight can be helped by glasses, though incipient disease may be responsible. After 60, however, most new disorders do not have a refractive origin, so that glasses are not the main form of treatment and the dangers of self-diagnosis increase.

Old people can fall into two groups in their attitude towards their eyesight. Either they fail to understand when no glasses can help them, or they accept failing eyesight as irremediable, even to the extent of not reporting it, especially to their doctor, who is not expected to be concerned with visual problems. Their relatives may adopt the same attitude. Fear of hospital deters many from following up their optician's advice to see their general practitioner. For this reason visual defects in the elderly must be searched for, rather as they are in children.

Much of the visual difficulty experienced by the elderly at home can be relieved by very simple means. The main aid is illumination. As the eye ages the pupil becomes more constricted, so that less light enters the eye. Because of this pupillary narrowing the elderly eye has a built-in gloom, which is seldom appreciated by others. About four-fifths of the deficit in light sense is attributable to this and can be restored by extra illumination.

## Reading difficulties: the commonest problem



The sight problems of old age are most commonly those of reading. Most old people, even those who are almost blind, can find their way round their familiar surroundings, although they become much more handicapped if they move, for example, to an old people's home. Their reading difficulties are with them wherever they are.

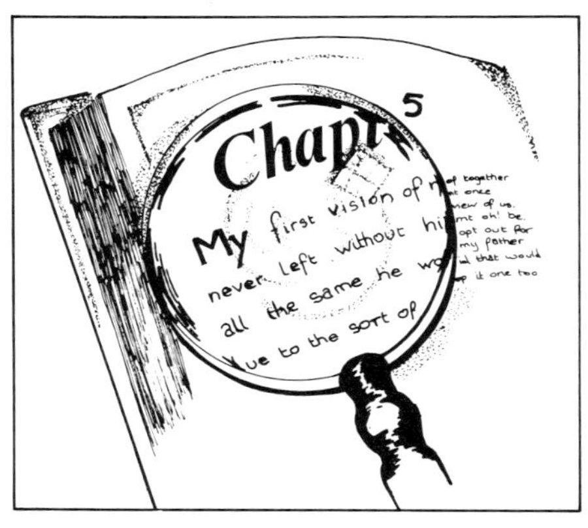

Some people can be helped by a hand or stand magnifying glass, but these are cumbersome to manage and all restrict the field of vision so that rapid reading is impossible. Telescopic lenses, whether for near or distant vision, have similar limitations but can be obtained on loan through the hospital eye service (though not through the optician or local ophthalmologist). Large-print books are available in public libraries, and books on tape or cassette can be obtained as a benefit by those who are certified as being unable to read.

The readability of print depends on both its size and contrast, black print on a white background being the easiest to read. In practice the importance of contrast is often not recognised. Government departments and other official organisations tend to forget this and print forms on buff or grey paper in coloured inks of poor density. Computerised or photocopied documents are often grey on grey.

## Eye and brain: both degenerate with age

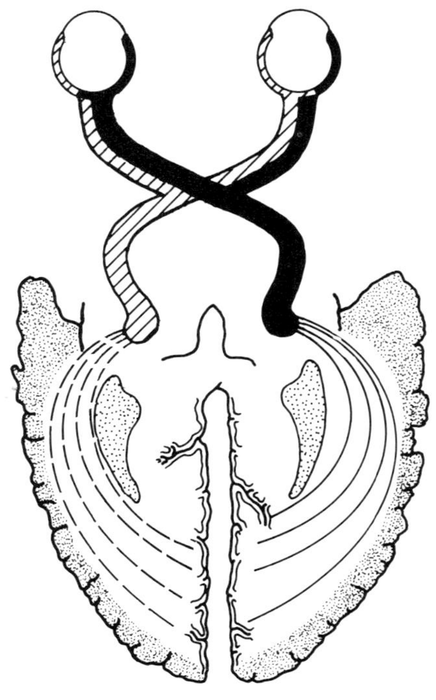

Sight depends on the eye and brain jointly. Many elderly people, particularly those with circulatory diseases, have degenerative changes in the nerve cells in the retina that primarily affect the macular area, whose health is necessary for seeing detail. At the same time similar cells in the brain deteriorate, or perhaps only the brain cells may be affected.

In the former group a confused brain is given the task of interpreting blurred images. These people are only slightly more handicapped than those whose eyes are normal but whose brains are not.

It is important to check the vision of the elderly at regular intervals because of the unpredictability of the rate at which visual loss may occur. All too often this requires elderly people to make great efforts to attend a hospital eye clinic, possibly by ambulance, where they are given a three-minute test and told that there is no change. Many default, with some justification, but need watching out for in their homes.

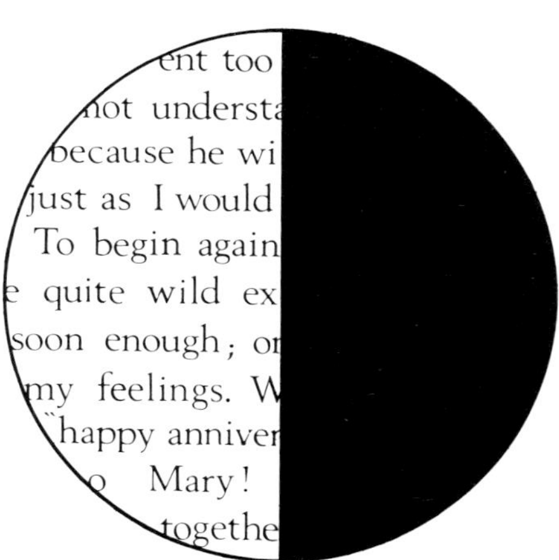

Victims of strokes are particularly hard hit and often have no insight into their condition. They commonly complain of their inability to read, and it may be hard to convince them, and sometimes their relatives, that they are on a false quest in trying to have something done to their eyes. The common loss of either the right or left half of the field of vision makes it difficult for them to follow a line of print. Many of these patients fail to describe their difficulty in reading. Little can be done to remedy these defects, but patients should be assured that they will not go completely blind and that it will not harm their eyes to use them.

The minority of old people who need eye surgery are often accorded a low priority on hospital waiting lists. The length of time on a waiting list is seldom related to life expectancy. For example, a 2-year-old child who has to wait two years for a non-urgent operation spends about two-seventieths of his life on the list. A person of 80 with a life expectancy of about five years will spend two-fifths of her remaining life on the same list. Very possibly she will have a worse prognosis after those two years. Old age itself might be a ground for priority if an operation is likely to transform a handicapped person into a more independent person. The general practitioner is in a position to point this out.

The section of the *Radio Times* was reproduced by kind permission of its editor.

# BLINDNESS AND PARTIAL SIGHT

## Loss of sight in one eye

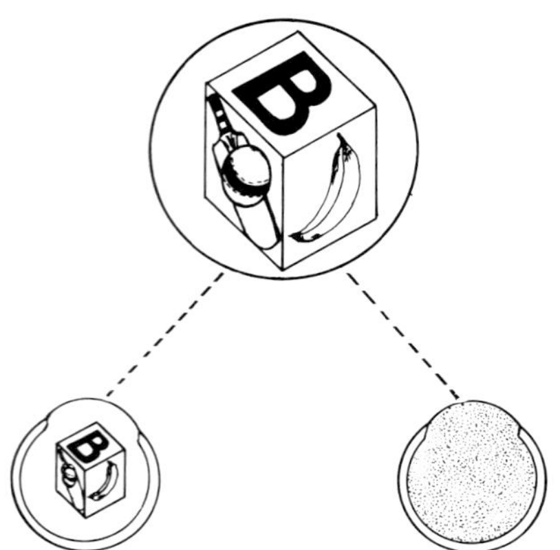

Losing the sight in one eye causes a handicap only to those who had good binocular vision or whose better eye is affected. The handicap in the previously binocular is difficulty with depth perception, which may preclude them from driving. Also, the loss of their accustomed field of vision may cause them to bump into things on one side.

Younger people usually adapt quickly to such difficulties. Those who have had sight in only one eye since infancy suffer no significant disability if the remaining eye is normal. Such people are not eligible for registration as partially sighted.

## Difficulty in reading

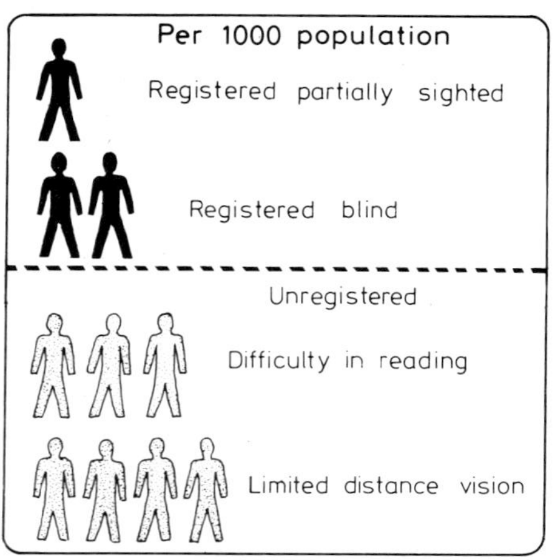


Difficulty in reading is obviously a handicap in education—more so than indifferent distance vision. But the criteria for establishing that someone is registrable as partially sighted and therefore has educational difficulties include no reference to near vision.

A survey carried out on the population of one English country town showed that 2 per 1000 people were registered as blind and a further 1 per 1000 registered as partially sighted. These figures corresponded to the numbers registered nationally but greatly underestimated the numbers of handicapped. A further 4 per 1000 had severely limited distance vision and 3 per 1000 had difficulty in reading. (T Cullinan, Health Services Research Unit Report No 28. Canterbury, University of Kent, 1977.)

Improved lighting is one major way of helping those with visual handicaps, and large-print books are available from public libraries. Unfortunately, government and other official forms do not come in large-print versions and the partially sighted often have to rely on others to fill them in.

## Blindness and partial sight



The visually handicapped are those whose sight with glasses is imperfect. The largest group is the elderly, but all age groups include people whose vision is limited because of congenital conditions, general or ophthalmic disease, or trauma.

These people receive social benefits if registered and are divided into two groups: the partially sighted and the blind. Most of those registered as blind can see, though not very well. Distance acuity of 3/60 or worse is the basic requirement, but field loss is also taken into account. Partial sight requires a visual acuity of 6/60 or less, but, again, field loss allows some flexibility.

The benefits of registration as a blind person include an extra tax allowance, a reduced TV licence fee, limited travel concessions, and access to talking books on tape. The Royal National Institute for the Blind will advise on aids such as guide dogs, long canes, etc. One survey of the registered blind showed that only half of them had received a visit from a social worker, this being no longer statutory.

An anomaly of the system is that those on the blind register pay a reduced TV licence fee, whereas those registered as partially sighted, who can usually see television but cannot see to read, do not qualify for this reduction. Special certification from an ophthalmologist is necessary for the partially sighted to receive talking books.

Registration is effected through the director of social services and requires a consultant's signature. It is not statutory but voluntary and can be a difficult topic to introduce to a patient if the word "blind" is used. Whenever possible the term "handicapped" should be used, which will avoid unnecessary fears of deterioration. This applies equally to infants and the elderly.

Anyone can paint a stick white and use it as a sensible precaution in busy streets and while crossing roads. All those with visual handicaps or concerned with the visually handicapped will be greatly helped by the BBC's "In Touch" programme and its booklet.

---

LARGE PRINT BOOKS :

     Public libraries and National Library for the Blind, 35 Great Smith Street, London SW1; 5 St John Street, Manchester.

TALKING BOOKS :

     British Talking Book Service for the Blind, Nuffield Library, Mount Pleasant, Wembley, Middlesex.

BRAILLE BOOKS :

     National Library for the Blind (for loans), Royal National Institute for the Blind, 224 Great Portland Street, London W1, Scottish Braille Press, Graigmiller Park, Edinburgh (publishers).

RADIOS :

     British Wireless for the Blind Fund gives radios on permanent free loan to registered blind people (apply through social services department).

TELEPHONES :

     Telephones for the Blind Fund, Mynthurst, Leigh, Nr Reigate, Surrey, may give help with installation or rental.

---

# Educating partially sighted children

Historically the partially sighted came to be recognised only because they were assumed to be on their way to blindness. Their registration was not to enable them to obtain benefits but to mark them out for special education or retraining if their occupation became impossible. Therefore only in the younger age groups is registration for partial sight worth while. There are special schools for these children, where their inability to read is catered for by the use of magnifiers and audiovisual techniques.

The difficulties for the partially sighted child in ordinary schools usually occur at about the age of 7, when the fluent reading of fairly small print is demanded. Special schools usually have a higher staff-pupil ratio than usual, have specialised equipment, and provide a more secure atmosphere for children who might feel self-conscious about their visual difficulties. Furthermore, most special schools have a visiting ophthalmologist who can help and support both children and staff. This is not the case when a visually handicapped child attends normal school. A disadvantage of special schools, especially when children board, is that they rarely mix with other children. The decision whether to send a child to a special school is usually best decided on the basis of an individual child's need rather than by reference to set visual standards. The present system for registering children leaves the final decision on schooling to the education authorities, and ophthalmic and medical statements are only one part of the total picture of the child's needs.

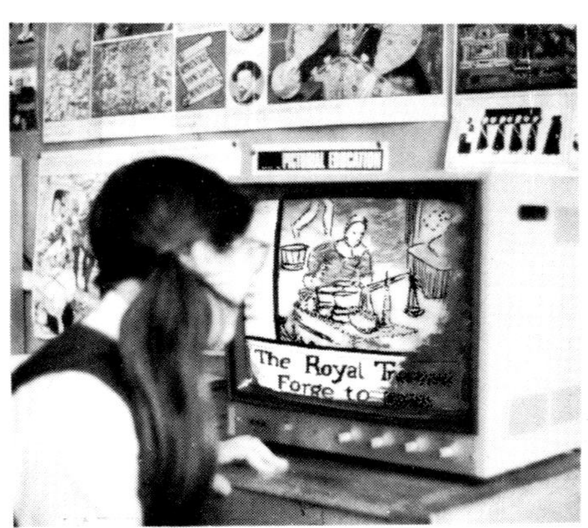


Closed circuit television at a school for the partially sighted

# The risk to future generations: genetic counselling

By school-leaving age children with a visual handicap should have been told whether they are likely to pass it on to future generations. This information should be totally reassuring to those with no hereditary condition, but children who have hereditary conditions should not be unduly alarmed. In many cases offspring will be affected only if both parents carry the gene responsible.

Sufferers from hereditary conditions—even such a well-publicised one as retinitis pigmentosa—cannot be advised except on an individual basis within a given family. In some there is a negligible risk of transmission, in others a very likely risk.

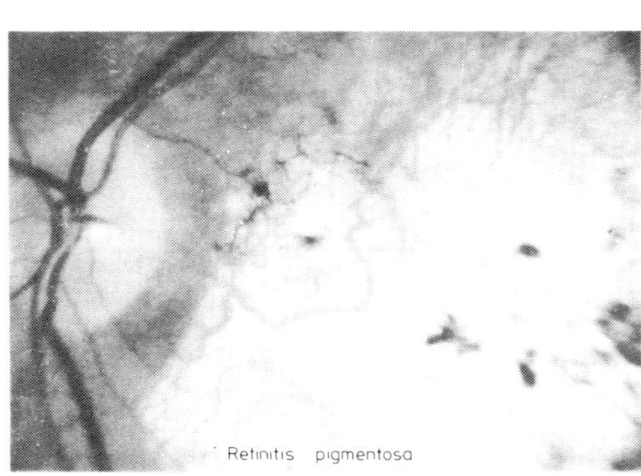

Retinitis pigmentosa

The photograph of closed-circuit television was reproduced by kind permission of Mr Bignall, headmaster of John Aird School, London; that of retinitis pigmentosa by permission of the Institute of Ophthalmology.

# OPHTHALMIC SERVICES IN THE NHS

## Ophthalmologists and opticians

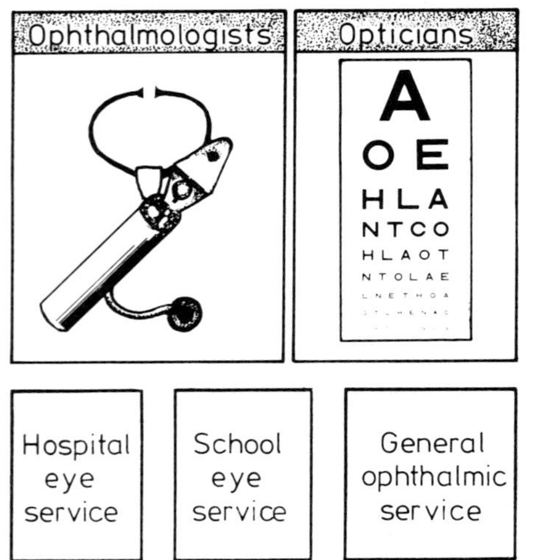



The ophthalmic services are broadly divided into two groups: the hospital-based services and the General Ophthalmic Service (GOS), which provides a service limited to sight testing (refraction) outside hospital. There is also special provision for schoolchildren, which is now under the community health services.

Specialists dealing with the care of eyes also fall into two distinct groups: those with medical qualifications and those without—ophthalmologists and opticians respectively.

Consultants in ophthalmology have to possess surgical qualifications. Most eye disorders, however, do not need purely surgical treatment, and many are part of diseases of a general medical or neurological nature. The consultant's professional life is therefore generally a blend of surgery, medicine, and refraction. Refraction is important because abnormalities obstruct normal function and its assessment.

There are also many other doctors practising full-time or part-time ophthalmology who have limited their activities by excluding surgery. The GOS, however, recognises only their ability to diagnose and does not permit them to treat outside hospital, except by prescribing glasses. Treatment other than glasses cannot be obtained under the GOS, though the general practitioner may, of course, treat eye disorders medically, with or without advice from an ophthalmologist. The result is that many patients with quite simple medical eye conditions are forced to visit hospital for treatment.

## General Ophthalmic Service

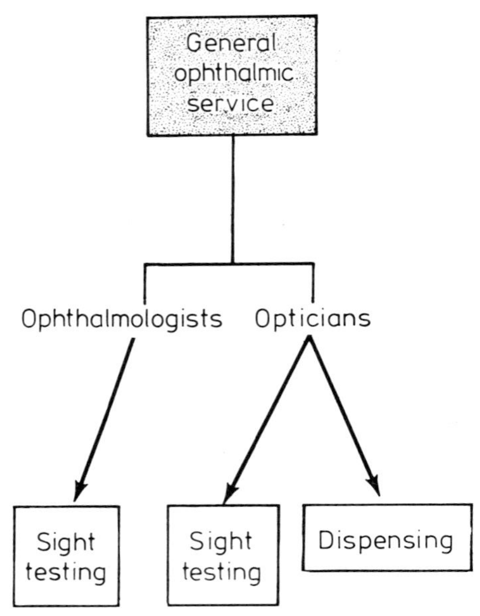



The GOS is essentially a sight-testing service and a system whereby the many people who self-diagnose the need for glasses can get confirmation that this is so or whether disease is present. It is manned by ophthalmologists who are often consultants doing part-time work outside hospital and by opticians who are either ophthalmic (sight testing) or dispensing.

A sight-testing optician's training is basically restricted to the optical functions of the eye and its disorders. Obviously this demands some knowledge of whether the eye is otherwise normal, but opticians are not qualified to diagnose or treat eye conditions. Their function is to improve acuity by providing glasses. If they suspect other abnormalities or cannot **improve defective vision they must refer patients to their general** practitioner.

It is often extremely difficult for doctors to identify a condition from the patient's complaints of discomfort. And it may be equally difficult for an optician to differentiate between an optometric condition and a medical condition which may represent a serious threat to eyesight. In addition patients are generally reluctant to tell opticians about their general health. Any information that passes either way is likely to be garbled by the patient. Comparatively few ophthalmic opticians are to be found in the hospital service or in community clinic work outside hospital.

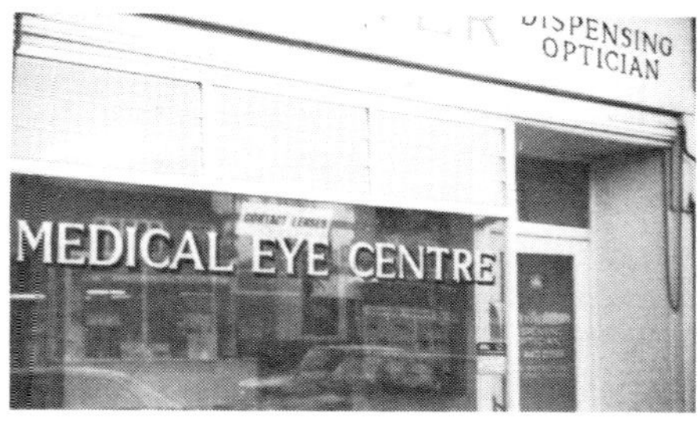

Dispensing opticians are qualified only to make and fit glasses to someone else's prescription. This skill is very important because inadequate fitting may itself undo any good the glasses were prescribed for—even to the extent of producing double vision, for example. Dispensing opticians often work in liaison with ophthalmologists and provide consulting rooms for them. These establishments are known as medical eye centres, where ophthalmic medical practitioners perform the refraction rather than sight-testing opticians, in many cases providing an indirect personal link with the hospital service.

## School eye service

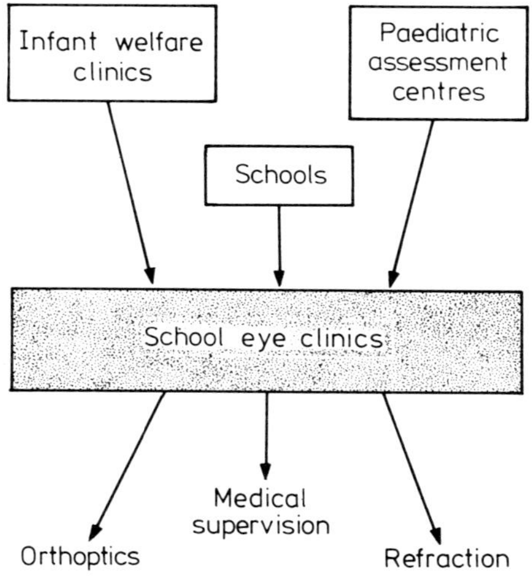


The school eye service was originally set up by local authorities to deal with the fact that neither children nor their parents notice or necessarily report their eye defects. Screening schoolchildren showed that many had poor vision and were unlikely to have anything done for them unless it was made easy. Clinics manned by ophthalmologists were therefore set up outside hospital, to which children were referred by the school doctor with the parents' agreement. These clinics opened the way to better medical treatment for squints, including the employment of orthoptists, and to the provision of medical opinion on the need for glasses and the role of eyesight in poor performance at school. (Prescriptions are issued under the hospital eye service, not the GOS.)

It gradually became apparent that screening at school entry was not early enough, so that children's eye services developed in some areas drawing patients from infant welfare clinics as well as from schools. Now community physicians have taken over the school medical service from local authority medical officers of health. Community physicians may have a greater role to play in catering for the diverse needs of the population for ophthalmic care, perhaps with the opening of developmental and geriatric clinics. Paediatric assessment centres, for example, often need ophthalmic opinions. The school eye service is excellent for detecting all children's visual defects by screening and following them up, neither of which is systematically dealt with by the hospital eye service or the GOS.

## Providing sight tests and glasses

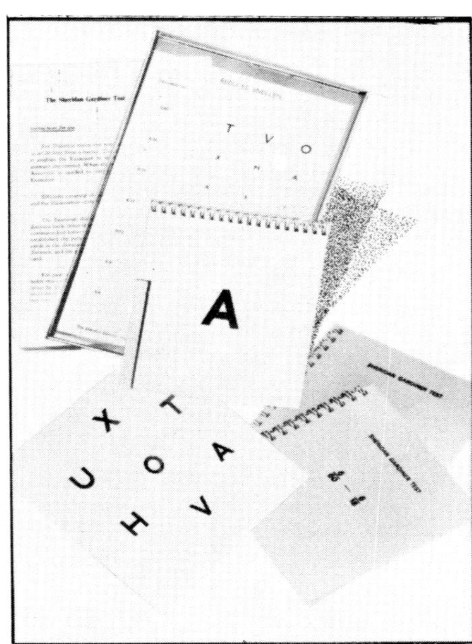

Sight tests are free under the NHS and can be obtained by anyone from birth onwards without medical advice or referral. If they are requested more than once a year by adults special circumstances must justify the test. A doctor's letter is usually accepted by the administration but referral for a second eye test is not desirable as a means of obtaining a second opinion, which is better obtained privately or by a hospital consultation under the NHS.

Children's sight may change within short intervals—3 to 6 months—and special regulations apply to their eye tests.

The accepted practice of having an eye test every two years is not medically inspired. Any adult with a sudden new visual disturbance should seek advice within days and those with a gradual increasing disturbance within weeks. Those who are satisfied that each eye is performing normally without change can wait indefinitely in safety unless there is a strong family history of visual defect and disease.

Schoolchildren get glasses at special rates, but charges in general depend on the source of the prescription. Prescriptions issued from hospital for spare pairs of glasses, toughened lenses for children, and magnifiers of any sort are honoured by the NHS but not so if written by the same practitioner in the GOS. The best buy is therefore a hospital prescription. Glasses prescribed for hospital inpatients are totally free, but elderly people often have to pay considerable sums for their glasses after surgery —for example, for cataracts—because they are no longer in hospital when the glasses are ordered.

The GOS is therefore an effective organisation where healthy people can obtain sight tests and glasses, but it is not as useful as it might be for diagnosis and treatment. It has special limitations in respect of the handicapped and housebound.

# Ophthalmic services in the NHS

## The orthoptist

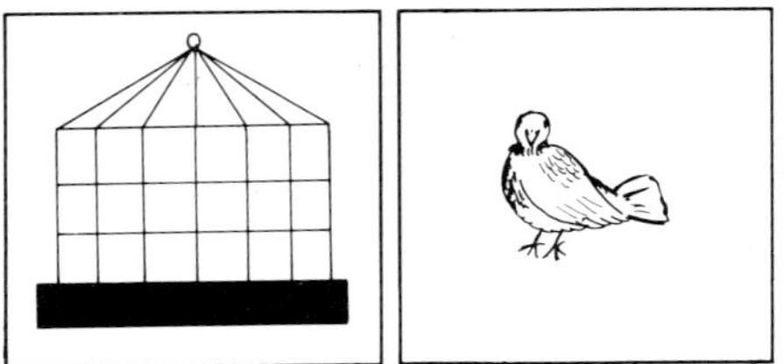

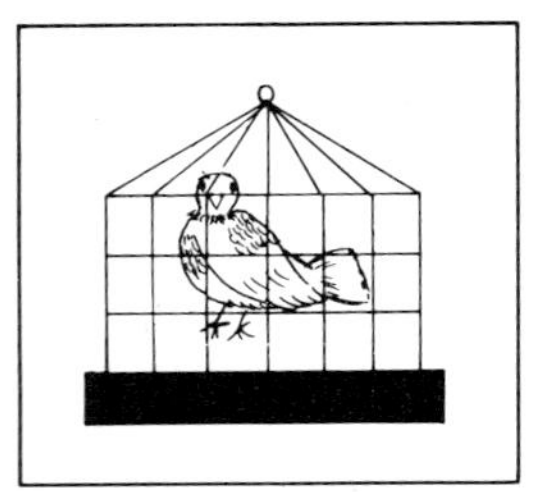

The orthoptist's work is similar to that of a physiotherapist: she is concerned with movements of the eye, in particular abnormal movements, which are mainly squints. Since squints are correlated with the development of visual acuity she is responsible, under an ophthalmologist, for supervising the treatment of children's eyes that are reluctant to play their full part in visual acuity or binocular vision. About 90% of the orthoptist's work is with children, mostly those aged under 7, but she has a useful role in the management of any disorder of binocular vision at any age. Such conditions include palsies or muscle imbalance, whether or not they are caused by trauma.

A newly squinting eye in an infant can lose its acuity in a few weeks, become conditioned to the abnormality, and build up secondary abnormalities in a few months that may take months or years to undo. Here the orthoptist has a valuable part to play in monitoring progress as well as in instituting actual treatment.

In most clinics orthoptists see only cases delegated for specific procedures, though in some areas they perform primary screening of children on behalf of the consultant and in others they see all doubtful cases of squint referred by GPs or from infant welfare clinics. Many combine hospital and school clinic work. Many attendances at orthoptic clinics over months or years are often necessary. Therefore this dispersal of the clinics is a boon to mothers who would otherwise default.

## Health visitors and social workers

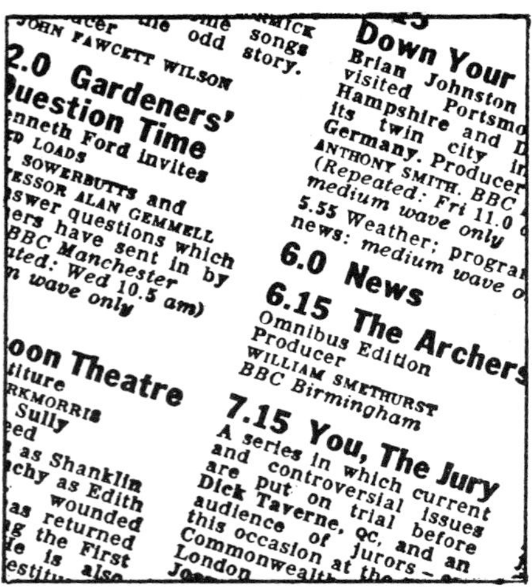

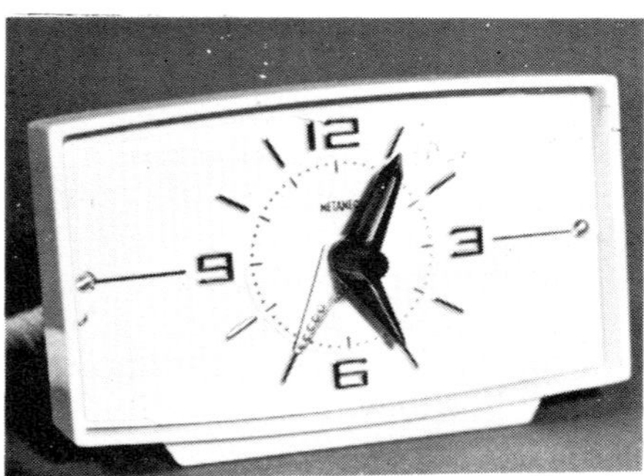

Alarm clock supplied by the Royal National Institute for the Blind

Both health visitors and social workers may be a great help to the visually handicapped. Health visitors, for example, are more likely to be asked about broken glasses or arranging a visit to an optician than doctors, and conversely, a health visitor can take an active role on her visits to the housebound. She may either ask direct questions about eyesight or do a simple reading test; the small print in the radio programmes is as good a test as any for reading difficulties.

Opticians have little inducement to visit people at home, which means there is a large gap in the services for the handicapped and housebound, though the general practitioner can always request a domiciliary visit from a consultant. The GOS rules apply to an optician's visit, but the more generous provisions of the hospital eye service are available through a consultant's visit.

Recent surveys in geriatric wards and at home have shown that not only do the elderly handicapped include many with defective vision but also that about 25% of the rational elderly are not getting theoretically easily obtainable remedies that would make life easier for them. This includes even some registered blind.

Social workers too should look out for visual problems and provide advice on help and aids. There are all sorts of aids for visually handicapped people. These include magnifying glasses, braille watches, extra illumination, telephone attachments, attachments for cooker dials, and so on. Problems to do with schooling and work often need sorting out.

Visual problems arise more often in children with other handicaps (physical or mental) than they do in normal children, and the social worker can legitimately inquire about eyesight at all ages and how any problems are being tackled. Social workers should not only be on the alert for people with visual handicap but also know whom to appeal to for practical and diagnostic aid. This is hard on the generic social worker, as the subject is so specialised.

The photograph of the Sheridan-Gardiner test is reproduced by kind permission of Keeler Instrument Ltd; that of the *Radio Times* by kind permission of its editor; and that of the alarm clock by kind permission of the RNIB.

# COMMON OR DIFFICULT DIAGNOSES

## Herpes ophthalmicus

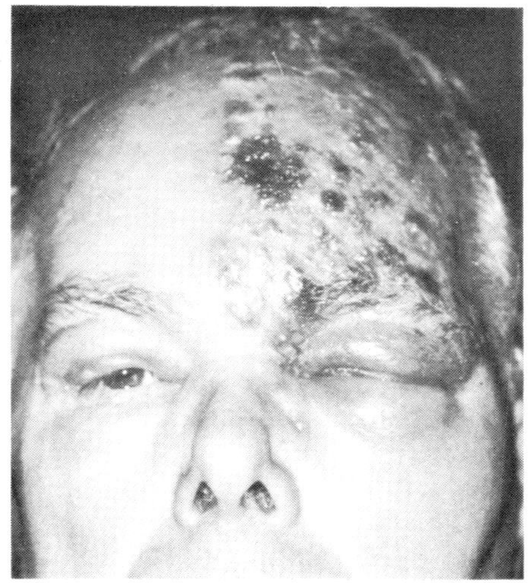

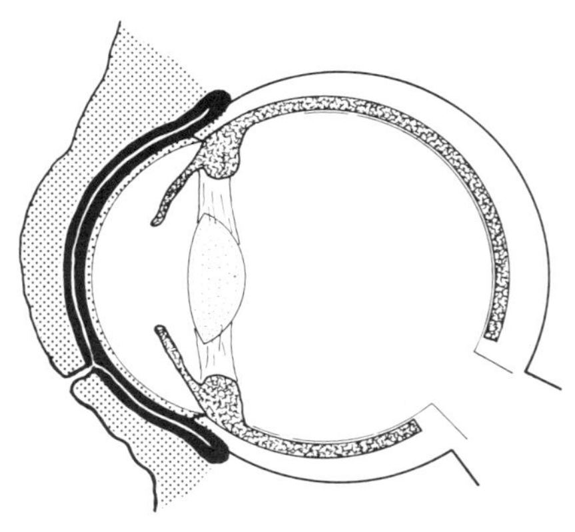


Herpes ophthalmicus (shingles) is caused by the same virus as chickenpox and may be acquired by chickenpox contacts. It is often misdiagnosed in its early stages and mismanaged in its later stages.

The first symptoms are numbness and tingling around the eye, followed in hours or days by redness and swelling of the lids. This swelling often prevents the opening of the lids, and the examiner might have great difficulty in separating them. These developments may be confused with an allergy. Pain and tenderness are usually severe.

The possibility of shingles may be rejected mistakenly because the disease seems to be spreading across the nose to the other eye, which is theoretically impossible for a process confined to the distribution of the fifth nerve. This is, however, never a true extension—merely a spread of oedema. A more common early complication is swelling and congestion of the conjunctiva. The oedema begins to resolve after a few days and the eye begins to open. The formation of skin vesicles may be early and gross or late and minimal.

On about the 10th to 14th day a quiet intraocular inflammation may begin, and the mild decrease in visual acuity that accompanies it is too often attributed to the violent storm that has occurred externally. If this inflammation is ignored serious complications and permanent visual handicap may result. The safest course is for all patients with shingles to have an ophthalmological opinion within a month of the first symptoms if they do not have completely normal near and distant vision. Acuity should, if possible, be tested at all stages.

The cornea often becomes anaesthetic: and keratitis is then a possibility; this may be potentially damaging to vision. Anaesthesia is not easy to determine when the lids are so swollen that the eye cannot be seen. But it should be tested by a wisp of cotton wool as soon as possible. If anaesthesia is present an ophthalmologist's opinion is needed within days.

Systemic analgesics may be helpful, but in all cases treatment of the conjunctiva with an antibiotic ointment will prevent secondary infection. Dusting powders help to dry out skin lesions. But the aftermath that afflicts so many patients is an intractable and often untreatable neuralgia. In some cases the cornea remains permanently anaesthetised, and this may warrant permanent protection against the elements or trauma; glasses with side shields are usually adequate.

## Conjunctivitis

Conjunctivitis in its common form is of infective origin and characterised by discharge as well as redness. Epidemics, though statistically recognisable, are of no great importance in temperate climates; in the tropics trachoma and ophthalmia neonatorum are still major causes of blindness. Normal hygiene is sufficient in the home without taking alarmist precautions against the spread of infection. Sensitivity to light is a common feature but it is no indication of severity or the presence of complications unless acuity is affected. Dark glasses may ease the discomfort, but on no account should the eye be covered.

If treatment is properly ordered and carried out most cases of infective conjunctivitis will improve within a few days and will have resolved completely in two weeks. Saline irrigations are helpful when discharge accumulates; and chloramphenicol drops every two to four hours, together with chloramphenicol ointment at night, will overcome the common organisms.

# Common or difficult diagnosis

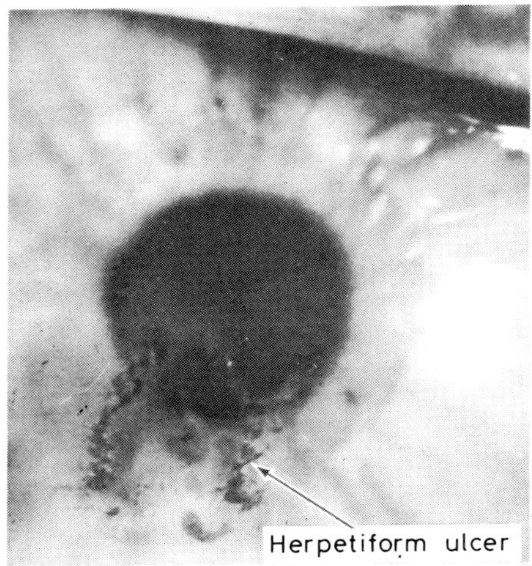

Herpetiform ulcer

If symptoms persist longer than two weeks, particularly if the onset of conjunctivitis was associated with evidence of a systemic viral disease such as influenza, there is a danger that some viral form of corneal damage is present. This is potentially far more dangerous than the conjunctivitis. There may be no more than minor redness but lacrimation is usually excessive. The damage can be detected by staining the cornea with fluorescein; under magnification the damaged area will appear coloured green.

In the early stages these herpetiform ulcers can usually be dealt with by outpatient treatment but they may become chronic and resistant later. Also the corneal opacification that results may cause some permanent visual loss.

Treatment includes firm padding and administration of idoxuridine drops 0·1% every hour with idoxuridine ointment every four hours. If no improvement occurs after 10 days of such treatment further advice should be sought. High doses of ascorbic acid for a few days encourage healing in many corneal conditions. In all cases of conjunctivitis steroid treatment is contraindicated.

## Allergies

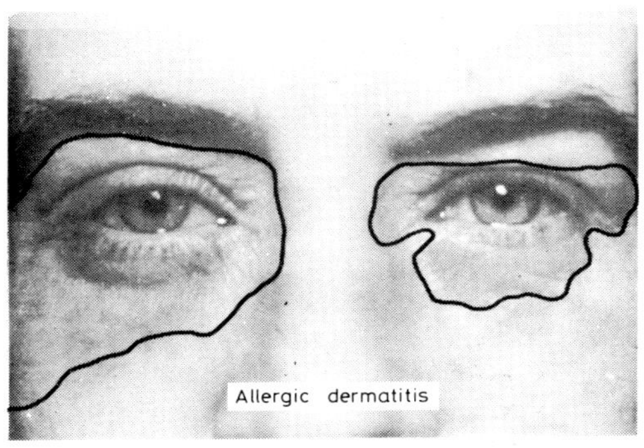

Allergic dermatitis

Many minor complaints which never impair vision are distressing and handicapping. True allergies include the irritable watering eye usually associated with catarrhal symptoms caused by pollen or other components of dust. Seasonal "hay fever" is the commonest form. Endogenous causes of this type of allergy are seldom found, but both endogenous and exogenous causes may produce the other common allergic dermatitis of the lids that shows itself not only by swelling of the lids but often of the conjunctiva too. Many of these patients suffer from the treatment given in an attempt to clear up the "conjunctivitis" that is thought to be the cause. People may be allergic to the antibiotic used or to the vehicle in which it is carried.

This is particularly so with ointments, where the base may be the agent. Some people, however, are allergic to the preservative in eye drops. Attempts to clear the condition by local treatment may be self-defeating. Stopping local treatment will then bring rapid relief, but the patient should be warned of the cause of the trouble as the susceptibility is longlasting.

Cosmetics and other chemicals, including detergents, may all cause allergic reactions. The eye reactions may be part of a more widespread allergic dermatitis. In all cases systemic antihistamine treatment is likely to bring relief.

## Lids: cysts, styes, and crusting

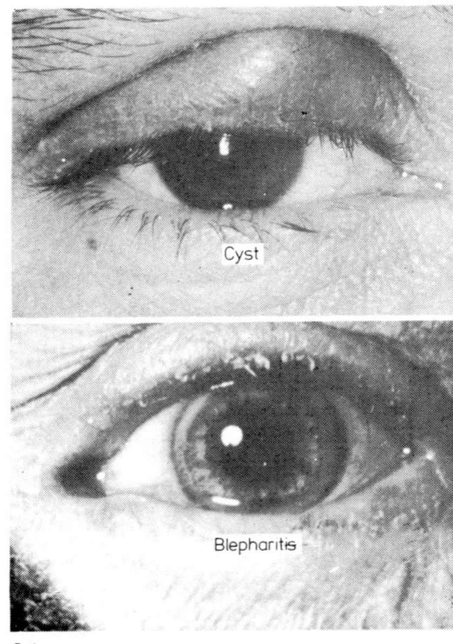

Cyst

Blepharitis

Cysts, styes, and crusting of the lid margins (blepharitis) are common. None are caused by using the eyes, but cysts on the upper lid may cause temporary visual defects. Cysts that do not resolve spontaneously need incision and dissecting out. Complications are virtually unknown. Any incapacity seldom lasts more than overnight.

Prolonged infective blepharitis in the days before antibiotics caused lid deformities and sometimes severe visual handicap from corneal damage and secondary infection. Local antibiotics usually control secondary infection. The underlying cause of blepharitis may be dandruff, which should also be treated. Congestion of the lid margins is often the precursor of blepharitis; it usually responds to hydrocortisone ointment, if only temporarily.

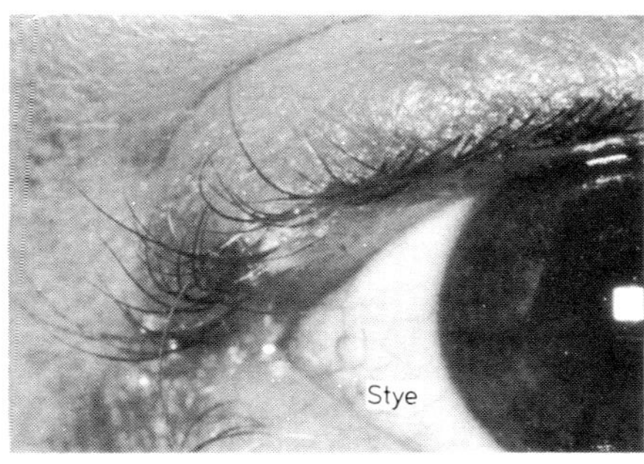



Styes (infections of the lash follicle) are no different from hair follicle infections elsewhere and have no relation to visual difficulties or any special significance in a healthy person. Most resolve spontaneously but this may be hastened by bathing with hot water, and removing a lash will sometimes encourage the abscess to drain. Systemic antibiotics should usually be avoided.

Recurrence, as in other parts of the body, may indicate a general lack of resistance, and treatment needs to be general rather than merely local.

The lids are also a favourite site for a rodent ulcer (basal cell carcinoma). Confirmation by microscopy is desirable. Any recurrent ulceration or induration of the skin should be excised or irradiated in its early stages, since delay may lead at best to more extensive surgery and at worst to such widespread and local extension that the ocular tissues are threatened.

## Lids: turning in or out

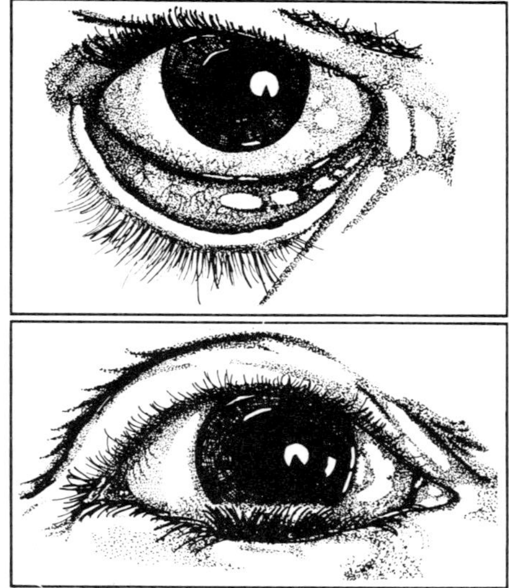

The lids may lose their ability to remain in contact with the globe. This usually happens to the lower lid as a result of injury or because of the degenerative changes of old age. The result is lacrimation and secondary infection. This may be potentially dangerous should the eye become diseased or need surgery for some other condition. Treatment should therefore be considered for what may appear to be a fairly trivial complaint.

If the lid falls away from the globe (ectropion) even to a minor extent watering will occur. Provided lacrimal drainage is intact this can be cured by simple plastic surgery as an outpatient.

When the lids turn in (entropion), the lashes scrape the globe. This often does not cause as much pain as might be expected, sometimes none at all, but the scraping can damage the cornea, threatening sight. Again simple plastic surgery is required. Turning in of the lid is often intermittent and may be missed.

## Cosmetic degeneration

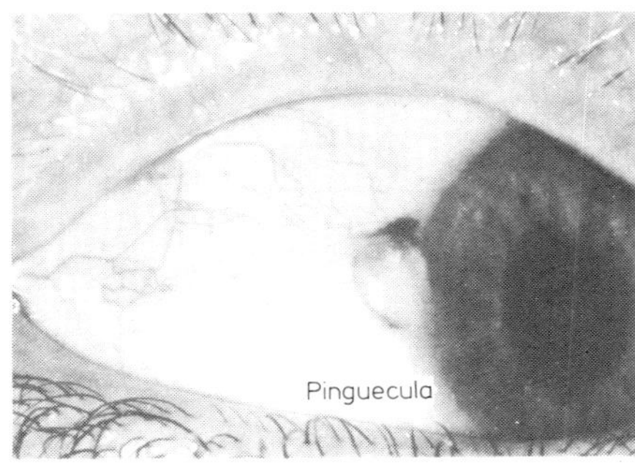



Those who are anxious about their appearance are often worried by what seem to be blisters or follicles or fatty deposits on the globe in the horizontal meridian (pinguecula). These are degenerative changes that have no pathological importance. Excision is seldom justified and not always successful in improving the appearance.

These should not be confused with the more serious slow-growing infiltration of the cornea (pterygium), starting from the point where it joins the sclera. In the UK it occurs only in people who have spent long periods overseas. In a few cases it may present a threat to sight. The infiltration may halt or it may take years to become serious. It needs removal for visual reasons only when it shows steady encroachment on to the cornea. Palliative treatment is useless and expert advice is needed once progression is observed.

The skin at the inner end of each lid is sometimes disfigured by fatty changes (xanthelamata). These are self-limiting, but often need excision for cosmetic reasons. They sometimes recur, though in people with raised blood cholesterol reducing the concentration may help. In the early stages this measure alone may cause slow spontaneous resolution.

Age is often accompanied by the appearance of a white ring around the edge of the cornea (arcus senilis). This is so common as to be physiological and never presents any threat to sight.

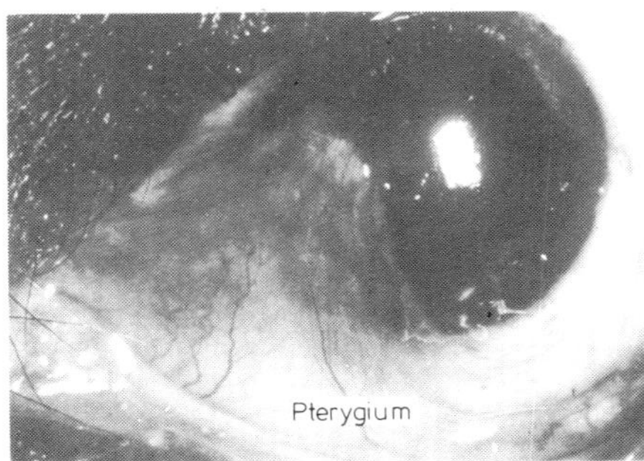



The photographs of herpes ophthalmicus, herpetiform ulcer, allergic dermatitis, cyst, blepharitis, stye, pinguecula, and pterygium were reproduced by permission of the Institute of Ophthalmology.

# EVALUATING COMMON SIGNS AND SYMPTOMS

## Visual symptoms always more serious

| | |
|---|---|
| Blurring | Lacrimation |
| Diplopia | Headache |
| Floaters | Pain and soreness |
| Nystagmus | Red eye |

In terms of function visual symptoms are always potentially graver than the non-visual ones, though to the patient discomfort in the eyes or noticeable redness may seem more serious.

## Blurring

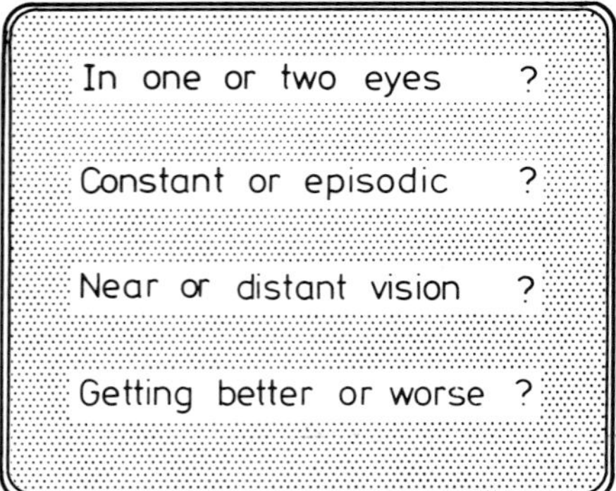


The commonest visual symptom is "blurring," which covers many meanings. To determine the importance of the blurring, the doctor must inquire whether it is equal in each eye or confined to one; constant or episodic; for near or distant vision, or both; of sudden onset; and whether it has changed since it was first noticed, and, if so, for better or worse. If the visual acuity can be established the severity of the disturbance will become much clearer.

Blurring in only one eye is much more likely to be ocular in origin than in both, especially if it is of sudden onset.

If the blurring has occurred gradually over months in both eyes in an otherwise healthy person, then the most likely cause is a change of refraction. In the elderly it may also be due to lens opacities if the blurring affects mainly distance vision, or to retinal circulatory disturbance if it affects mainly near vision.

A test with a card pierced by a pinhole will show whether or not the blurring is caused by refractive changes. If these are the cause then the visual acuity will improve when the patient looks out through the pinhole, placed close to his eye. This test will determine whether or not glasses are likely to solve the problem and therefore the person to refer the patient to.

If the blurring is of sudden onset—in weeks or days—in only one eye then it is certainly not refractive. Even so, a complaint of sudden onset may mean only that a long-standing defect has just been noticed. It is safest to assume, however, that the event is potentially serious and urgent unless it suddenly recovers. If it does recover and the person is healthy then waiting for a further attack before referring the patient to an ophthalmologist is justifiable.

If the blurring steadily gets worse day by day or week by week—even if it is only by minor stages—then the position is correspondingly urgent.

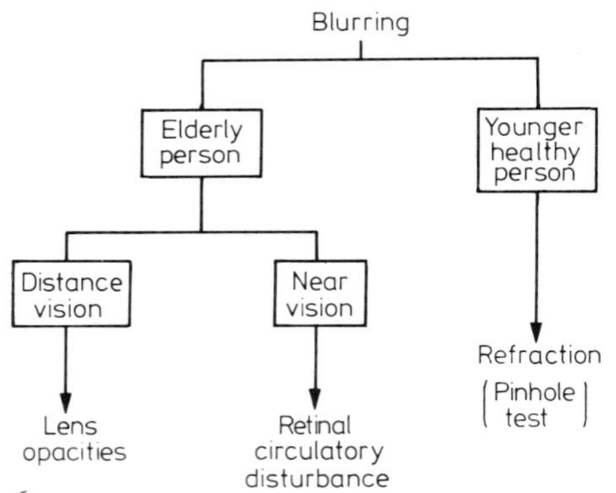

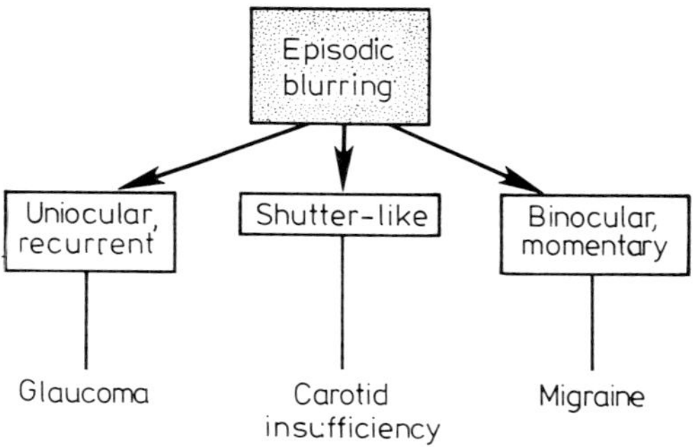



Episodic blurring (apart from that caused by changes in the light) is never due to a refractive error. If it occurs more than once a week in an adult over 35 there is a definite possibility of glaucoma, especially if it is uniocular and more than momentary. Multiple sclerosis is one of many causes of uniocular blurring lasting days or more.

Migranous episodes usually affect both eyes and occur for the first time in younger people. More rarely the episode of blurring may be caused by carotid insufficiency or its variants, and this is usually described as a shutter or blind effect.

# Diplopia

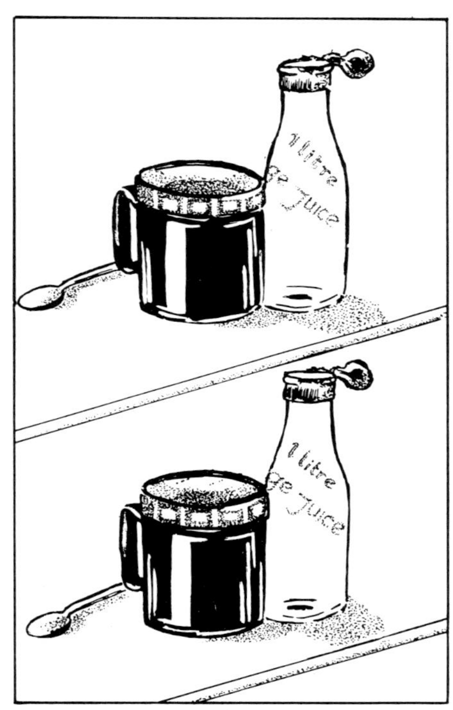



Double vision needs to be confirmed, as many patients confuse blurring or overlapping with double vision. True double vision means two separate objects—side by side or one above the other. There are three common causes of double vision in adults.

Firstly, paralysis or weakness may affect one or more of the extraocular muscles. The paralysis may be caused by trauma; local or intracerebral vascular lesions; idiopathic neuropathy, usually but not always associated with systemic conditions; multiple sclerosis; thyroid disease; myasthenia gravis; and diabetes. In all these conditions double vision may be the presenting symptom, and a tentative diagnosis may often be made by looking for the appropriate signs elsewhere.

Secondly, the eyes may intermittently fail to co-ordinate. This is a classic indication for orthoptic advice, possibly leading to the prescription of glasses or surgery. Young children will rarely complain and soon learn to suppress one image. In older people intermittent double vision might occur when they are under stress or sedation. Exercises may be needed to restore full function. Sometimes prismatic lenses solve the problem.

Thirdly, the angle of a long-standing squint may change. This is one of the difficulties of treating squints in adults. Squints should be treated in early life, when unwanted images can be suppressed.

# Floaters and blurred spots

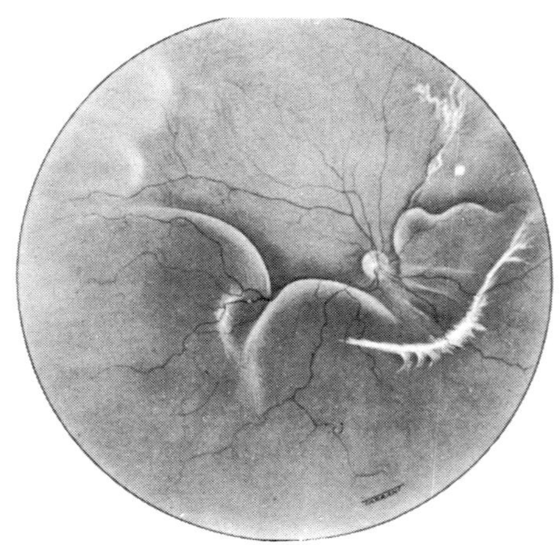

Retinal detachment

Perhaps the most common complaint after blurring is of spots floating about in front of the eyes. They may be one of the first signs of failing vision, especially in people with myopia, arteriosclerosis, or diabetes.

Floaters usually appear for the first time or are noticed for the first time when people are suffering from extreme fatigue or debility. The week or two after their onset is the critical time. If no further developments occur during this time, no serious changes are likely to occur if the visual acuity remains as good as it was. Any sudden change in acuity or in visual field in a short-sighted person may indicate a detached retina, especially if the spots are associated with seeing sparks or stars. The outlook in retinal detachment is improved greatly if the patient is treated immediately by an ophthalmologist. Floaters are more easily seen by the patient against a white background.

Circulatory disturbances in the retina may also cause bouts of seeing stars or flashes, particularly in the temporal field at times of fatigue or stress. These seldom forecast visual changes in the elderly if they are unaccompanied by floaters, and it is safe to await developments for a while in people with known arteriosclerosis or hypertension if acuity is unaffected.

# Evaluating common signs and symptoms

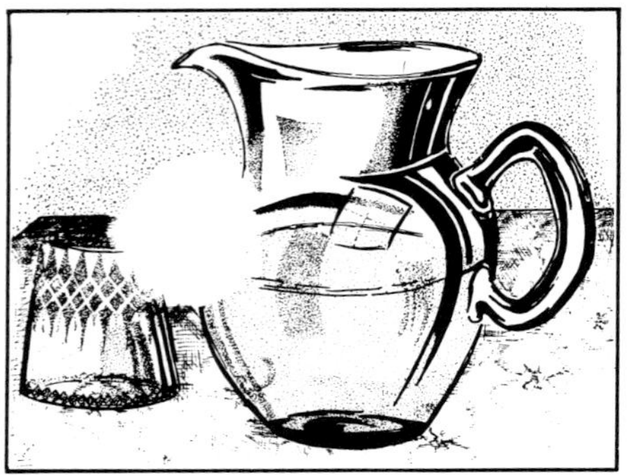

Floaters must be distinguished from the much rarer solitary area of blurring that does not float but moves with the eye without any time lag. This may be described as a piece missing from an object or a blurred spot and it tends to be constantly present. They are more serious than the common floater because they are often progressive or indicative of some other disorder, such as retinal disorders and neurological and cerebral conditions.

## Measuring acuity as a guide to urgency

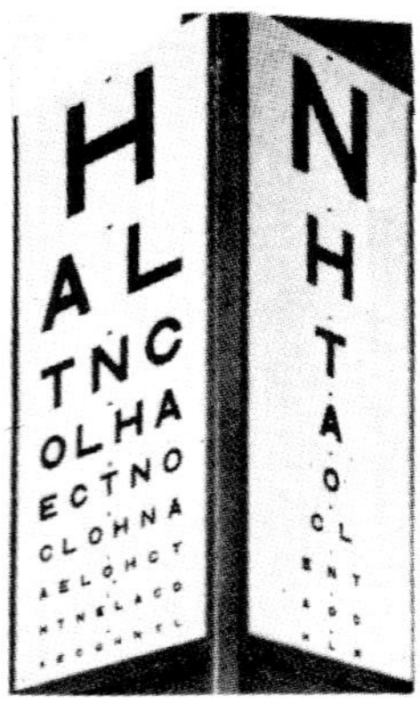

The actual measurement of visual acuity is the surest guide to changes that need investigation soon and those that can wait. The recorded loss of one line on the standard sight testing chart is sufficient warning if of recent onset.

The family history should influence the interpretation of these symptoms. But the patient is also guided by the family history and may jump to conclusions and either produce a symptom to fit a traditional history or suppress the history through fear.

The possibility that some of these purely visual symptoms may be the presenting symptoms of systemic disease must not be overlooked. Anaemia, for example, may present with only visual symptoms, the cause of which lies entirely outside the eye, and there are many others.

## Pain



Visual disturbance with pain *in* the eyes is always serious, and advice is urgently needed. Such conditions include iritis, glaucoma, multiple sclerosis, shingles (in which pain predominates late in the disease and disfigurement and swelling in the early stages), cranial arteritis, and sometimes hysteria.

An ingrowing eyelash may also cause pain in the eye—that is, somewhere inside the lids—as may more serious trauma, though this tends to be associated also with redness and watering.

A painful white eye with no visual symptoms is more likely to have a neurological basis than an ophthalmological one—for example, trigeminal neuralgia.

## Soreness



Symptoms of grittiness and hotness are common in middle age, but little is understood about how these are caused in the absence of visual disturbance. Nobody with an uncomfortable eye is going to lose their sight for that reason alone. These symptoms tend to be more common in women than in men and are almost always bilateral.

Some people who suffer sore or irritable eyes are the victims of an allergy —sometimes to an eye ointment. But one of the commonest causes of soreness and grittiness without visual symptoms is subclinical diminution in lacrimation. This is extremely common in people with arthritis, and will be aggravated in hot dry atmospheres.

Artificial tear drops often help more than over-the-counter eye lotions. If these fail and no other cause is found for the soreness, the patient may at least be assured that it is not a sign of approaching visual failure. Refractive disorders are seldom relevant.

# Lacrimation

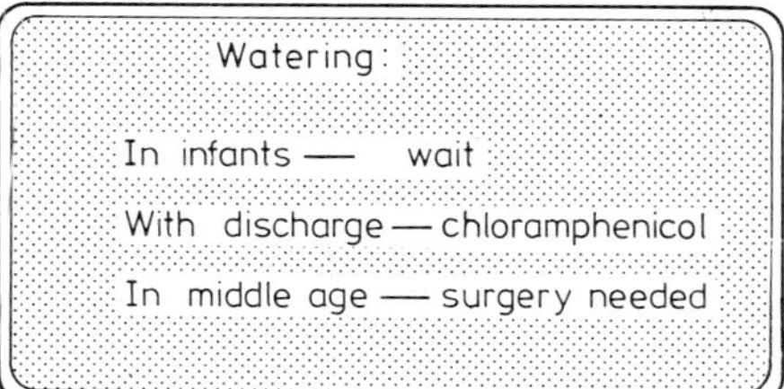



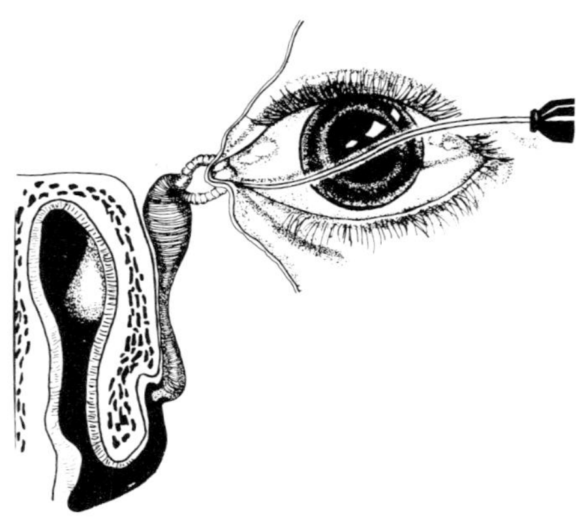

Lacrimation in a white painless eye is commonly found in infants and in the middle-aged and elderly. If it is unaccompanied by discharge it has no importance but may be intractable. In infants lacrimation tends to clear by 9 months because it is caused by delayed canalisation of the nasolacrimal duct. Since treatment necessitates a general anaesthetic and mechanical probing of the duct, delay while nature does its work is the better course. Watering alone has no implications for sight. Watering accompanied by discharge requires treatment with chloramphenicol ointment or drops, and if the discharge is resistant referral is indicated after two or three weeks.

In middle age, on the other hand, delay of months in probing or syringing often makes reconstructive surgery of the duct necessary. Delay may also lead to abscess formation, though this is less common now that antibiotic treatment is available.

If the lacrimal duct is patent lacrimation is commonly caused by loss of tone in the eyelids, or spasms of the lower lid leading to eversion or inversion, particularly in the elderly. This is simply remedied by minor outpatient surgery. Once again, a fine ingrowing eyelash may be a single cause.

In younger people (particularly students) excessive watering might be caused by the eyes' inability to converge without effort. The patient usually describes it as watering when he is reading or trying to read. It has nothing to do with refraction and the remedy is in the hands of the orthoptist. Lacrimation accompanied by pain or photophobia, on the other hand, may indicate corneal disease and is more serious (see below).

# Headache

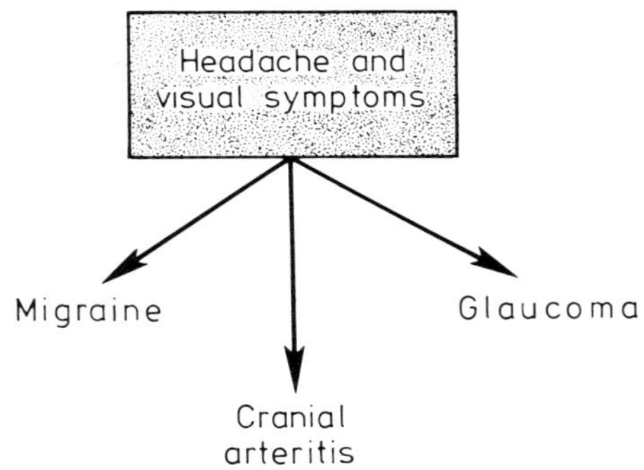



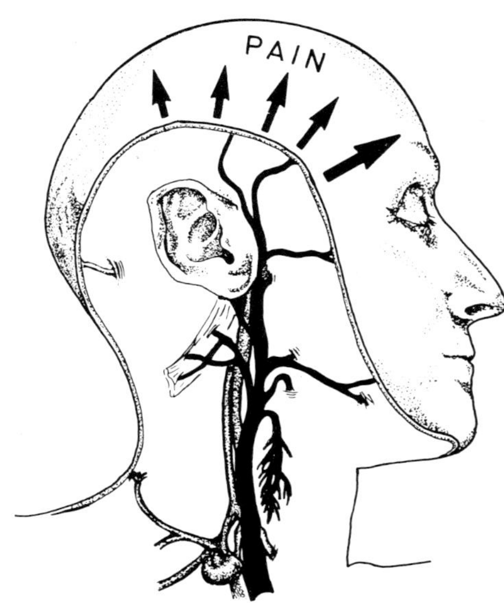



It is part of medical folklore that the eyes play an important part in producing headaches. An "eye check" is often therefore one of the first eliminating rounds in making a diagnosis.

Headaches that are not associated with visual symptoms or use of the eyes do not primarily need visual treatment or investigation: the cause of the headache must be sought elsewhere.

Even in people with headache and visual symptoms, ophthalmic treatment is not always indicated—for example, in migraine. The medical history should give a clue but a common error is to mistake the jazzy coloured aura of migraine for the rainbow seen by patients with glaucoma. The fact that glaucoma is rare before the age of 40 should help diagnosis in younger people. The migrainous spectrum is a spontaneous, jagged, firework-like phenomenon rather than the steady coloured illusion produced by a light source that is typical of glaucoma.

The glaucomatous headache usually occurs only while the blurring of vision is present, and it is seldom severe: it is often also accompanied by aching of the eye. In neither case is an eye test the sensible step. Patients with migraine need a physician and those with glaucoma an ophthalmologist.

Neither of these headaches need instantaneous treatment, but the headache of cranial arteritis does, as it may cause blindness in 24 hours. The headaches of arteritis always occur in the elderly; they are severe and often diffuse. Temporal tenderness is only one manifestation. They are usually severe enough to be troublesome at night and hinder sleep.

In all these conditions the retina and optic nerve may appear normal.

Headaches of visual origin are extremely rare in children aged under 10. They are also rarely caused by refractive disorders in children.

# Evaluating common signs and symptoms

## Giddiness and nystagmus

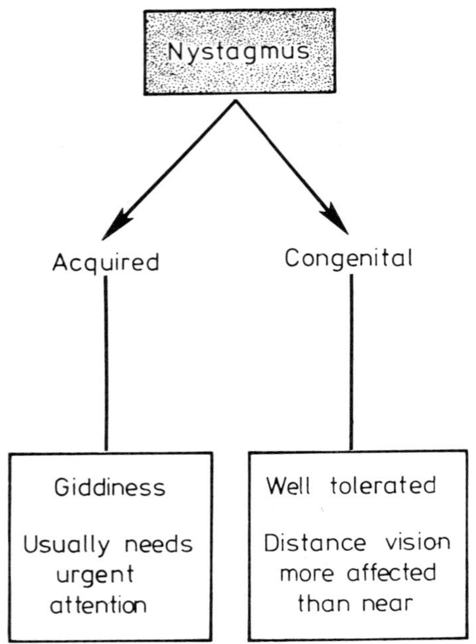



Giddiness, though sometimes associated with abnormal eye movements is seldom caused by a primary ocular disorder. Uncertain orientation may, however, be caused by sudden loss of sight in one eye, sudden loss of visual field (usually in cerebrovascular disease), or by variable diplopia of recent onset badly described. The cause is often neurological—for example, multiple sclerosis.

Whenever dizziness is reported information on eye movement is very useful because double vision might be confused with giddiness.

In congenital nystagmus the symptoms will be those of a well-tolerated defect. Visual acuity is always affected more for distance than for near sight, though a change in head posture may enable normal acuity to be obtained. After the age of 3 the defect usually becomes static, hence the toleration. The underlying cause is not understood but developmental ocular anomalies are common and often causal—for example, albinism—colobomata.

In acquired nystagmus giddiness may be the predominant complaint, though it may be noticed only under certain conditions. Whether the giddiness causes the nystagmus or vice versa depends on where the disturbance originates.

Acquired nystagmus elicited with or without accompanying symptoms is likely to be of urgent importance. Among possible causes are cerebral tumours, multiple sclerosis, and disorders of ear or labyrinth.

## Red eye: acuity more important than colour

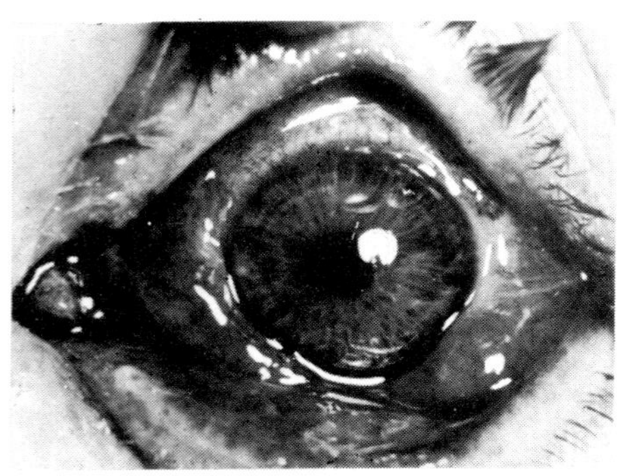

A red eye is not necessarily more serious than a white one. Once again it is the visual acuity that matters, but red eyes are not cured by correct refraction.

If any visual disturbance, however slight, accompanies the redness, a firm diagnosis is needed from an ophthalmologist within days, unless the eye and its acuity steadily improve.

The depth and extent of the discoloration are no guide to the severity of the condition. A spontaneous subconjunctival haemorrhage that totally obliterates the white sclera, is, in the absence of trauma, harmless and carries no complications. It will resolve on its own without treatment. On the other hand, redness in one eye that is hardly noticeable may signal intraocular disease and a potential threat to sight. Most of the serious causes of red eye do not affect both eyes at once, so uniocular redness is generally more of a danger signal than binocular redness.

For example, true infective conjunctivitis is usually binocular and not usually a serious disease in Western countries. The fact that there is always some discharge in conjunctivitis (which might be so slight that it only makes it hard to separate the lids on waking) distinguishes the condition from other causes of red eye. Treatment of a discharging eye can be safely left to local antibiotics for a week or so, but failure to respond in this time may well indicate corneal complications, especially if the patient has been suffering from a systemic or local virus disease. Permanent visual loss is a real possibility in such cases. Staining with fluorescein will show this under magnification.

The practice of covering red eyes is fortunately dying out, since covering an infected eye incubates the organism, hinders recovery, and may spread the infection.

The conjunctivitis and other signs of ocular irritability that accompany measles have no special significance.

It is important to distinguish infective or viral conjunctivitis from other forms of red eye because steroid treatment is contraindicated in conjunctivitis.

Any of these symptoms occurring in a person with only one useful eye warrant a completely different scale of urgency about referral than if they occur in one of a pair.

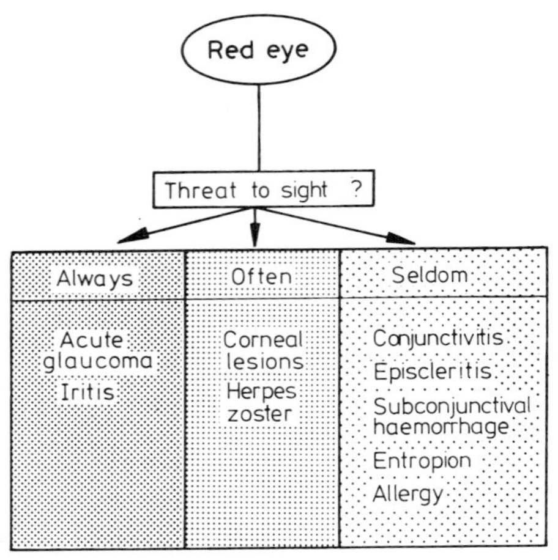



The photographs of retinal detachment and red eye were reproduced by permission of the Institute of Ophthalmology; that of an eye chart by kind permission of Keelers Instruments Ltd.

# GENERAL MEDICINE AND VISUAL SIDE EFFECTS

## Blurring: the major presenting symptom

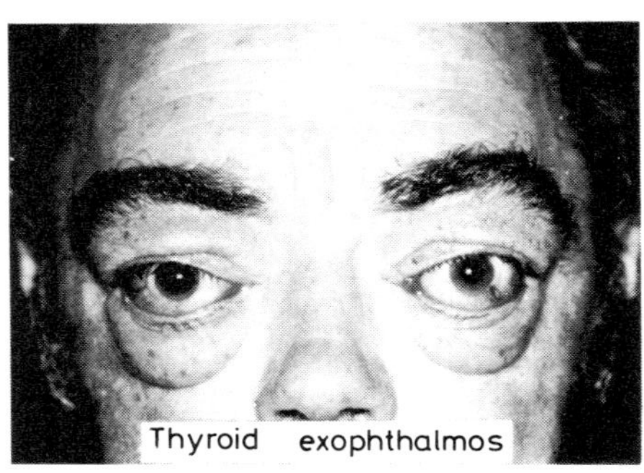
Thyroid exophthalmos

Many general diseases may affect the eye or present with ocular signs (see list). For example, thyroid disease may present with double vision as the primary complaint, and many of the collagen diseases present primarily with eye signs. Conditions such as Still's disease, spondylitis, and other rheumatoid conditions may be heralded by visual changes caused by uveitis and choroiditis.

Nearly all the ocular conditions mentioned are described by the patient as blurring of vision—if they are mentioned at all. Patients often think that eye disorders are a natural expectation in the course of a general disease. Therefore thorough case-history taking should include a specific reference to vision. Many of these conditions are potentially blinding if unrecognised and untreated.

| Disease | Common ocular manifestations |
| --- | --- |
| Acne rosacea | Corneal vascularisation and ulceration |
| Anaemia | Ocular muscle imbalance, intraocular haemorrhages |
| Ankylosing spondylitis | Intraocular inflammation (uveitis) |
| Carotid insufficiency | Transient visual loss |
| Cerebral arteriosclerosis (stroke) | Field loss, visual agnosia |
| Cervical sympathetic malfunction | Drooping lid, small pupil, retraction of globe (Horner's syndrome) |
| Cranial arteritis | Sudden permanent loss of vision, cataracts, intraocular haemorrhage, retinal disease |
| Diabetes | Cataracts, intraocular haemorrhage, retinal disease |
| Multiple (disseminated) sclerosis | Nystagmus, double vision, visual loss |
| Facial palsy | Lid closure fails, lacrimation, corneal damage |
| Gonorrhoea | Conjunctivitis, iritis |
| Herpes zoster | Pain and swelling of lids and conjunctiva, corneal damage, intraocular inflammation |
| Hypertension | Variable visual loss—intermittent or permanent |
| Maternal rubella | Congenital cataract, microphthalmos |
| Myasthenia gravis | Transient or recurrent double vision |
| Rheumatic diseases | Sore, dry eyes, iritis, episcleritis (post uveitis) |
| Sarcoidosis | Conjunctival nodules, uveitis |
| Sinusitis | Orbital pain, protrusion of globe, double vision |
| Thyroid disease (excess) | Protrusion of globe, double vision, corneal ulceration |
| Thyroid disease (deficiency) | Mild swelling of lids |
| Trigeminal neuralgia | Pain in and around eye and orbit |
| Trigeminal neuralgia (treatment of) | Anaesthetic cornea |

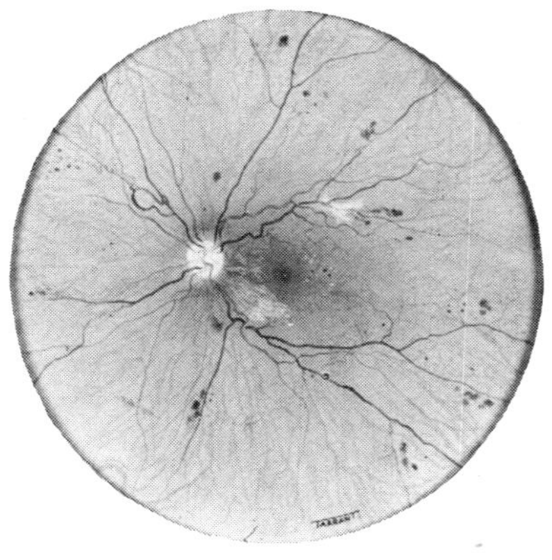

Diabetes deserves special mention. Its ocular complications occur earlier if it is inadequately controlled. Nevertheless, even if it is properly controlled the longer a patient has been diabetic the more likely visual symptoms are. Young diabetics are therefore more likely to suffer serious visual disorders eventually and need watching more closely than those with maturity-onset diabetes. Transient visual difficulties often occur during stabilisation.

# General medicine and visual side effects

## Iatrogenic disorders

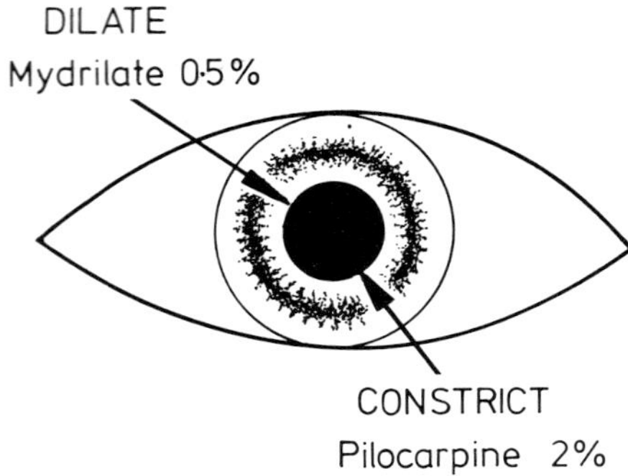



There are two main types of iatrogenic conditions. Firstly, those caused by local treatment and, secondly, those caused by systemic treatment of other diseases.

Apart from allergies to local treatment and the abuse of steroid drops, uncontrolled dabbling with pupil size can be hazardous. If the pupil is dilated with a weak mydriatic for examination it should always be restored to normal by a constrictor immediately after the examination; 2% pilocarpine is suitable. In older people a dilated pupil may cause a dangerous rise in intraocular tension, if it is not neutralised. A constricted pupil is not in itself dangerous, though it may exacerbate some conditions, such as iritis or uveitis. Atropine cannot be simply neutralised, and if it is applied locally to examine the eyes of young children it may cause hallucinations and nightmares.

The side effects of treatment of systemic diseases—for example, the ocular effects of practolol—are true hazards.

The risk of visual impairment by general treatment is exemplified by the use of life-saving oxygen in the newly born. Oxygen in high saturation used to be given without monitoring to premature babies, but it was later found to cause blindness. The lesion (retrolental fibroplasia) still occurs because of the choice at birth of "hyperoxygenation" or death in some cases.

The full list of drugs that may have visual effects is daunting (see Appendix). In general, visual complications of drug treatment tend not to arise in children or young adults, so the problem is one of middle and old age. Nearly all these drugs produce, among other effects, blurring of vision; this is serious only when it is irreversible. In people being treated with any of these drugs, medical ophthalmological advice should be sought if any visual symptoms occur, rather than look for better glasses.

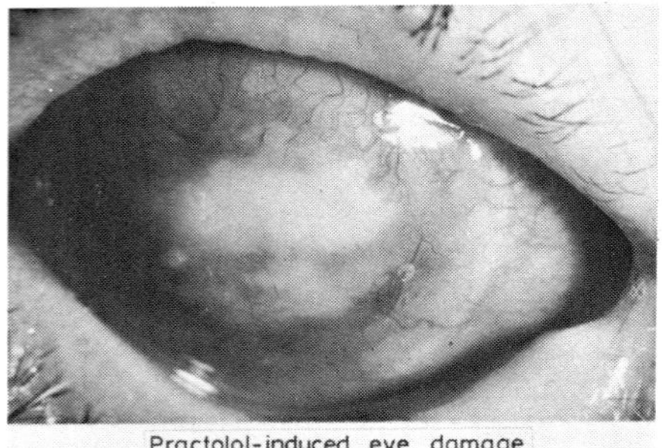

Practolol-induced eye damage

## Patients with unsuspected glaucoma most at risk

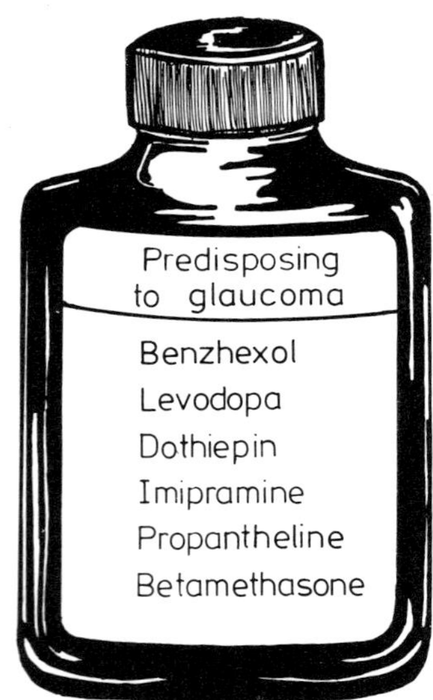



The patients who most commonly suffer are those with undiagnosed or incipient glaucoma, which may be precipitated or aggravated by drug treatment, especially in those with a family history. The drugs that most commonly precipitate glaucoma are anticholinergic preparations, especially those containing atropine or hyoscine. These drugs are mainly used for alimentary antispasmodics, in Parkinsonism, asthma, and travel sickness. Single-dose use, such as before an operation, is unlikely to provoke more than transient visual symptoms.

The middle-aged and elderly with chronic disease and receiving long-term treatment are those most at risk. They are also least likely to mention new visual symptoms, because they assume it is part of the disease or that something is wrong with their glasses.

Some of the drugs are safe in narrow-angle as opposed to wide-angle glaucoma and others the reverse, so it is best to ignore this distinction and seek an ophthalmological opinion when in doubt.

Any drug that is contraindicated in glaucoma should also be considered to be contraindicated in those who are predisposed to glaucoma. Preoperative injections of atropine may also be unwise in such people.

## Steroids

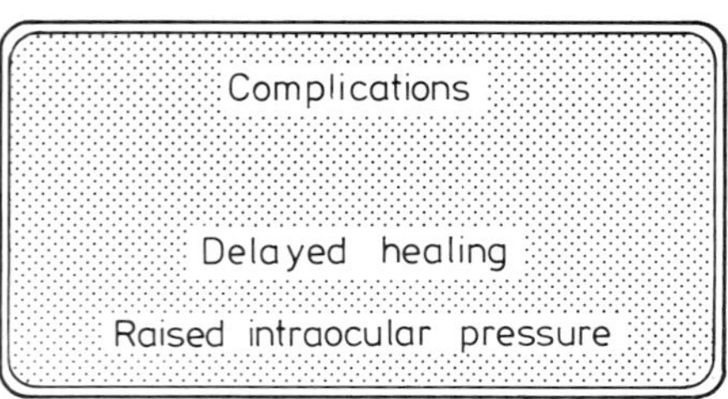



Locally steroids are extremely valuable, but they carry the risk of delaying healing, particularly of corneal lesions of viral origin. It is therefore unfortunate that so many local preparations should combine steroids with antibiotics. The use of steroids locally or systemically may increase intraocular pressure, so they should not be used in people who already have raised tension without collaboration with an ophthalmologist.

The clinical evidence that long-term treatment with systemic steroids causes cataracts is tenuous, and need not be the decisive factor in deciding whether to continue treatment. Nevertheless, once lens opacities have formed, yearly (or more frequent) ophthalmological surveillance is needed.

# Chronic disease: long-term treatment

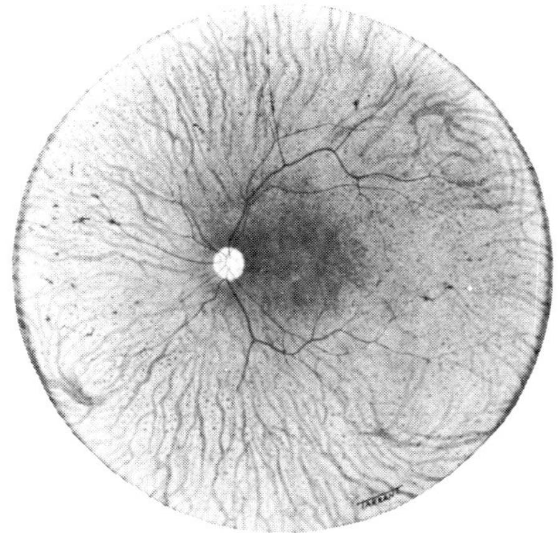

Chloroquine retinopathy

Chloroquine and similar drugs for malaria and liver abscesses are seldom used long enough for visual problems to arise. When their use is contemplated for longer periods, however, as in rheumatoid arthritis, irreversible damage may occur to the retina. Ophthalmological advice is essential in the event of visual symptoms and sensible before starting treatment.

Ethambutol is another drug which used long term is very likely to produce visual disturbance and possibly permanent visual loss due to a toxic effect on the retina. One difficulty that arises in chronic conditions where treatment is prolonged is that of assessing cause and effect. Most people on long-term treatment for conditions such as rheumatoid arthritis are of an age when degenerative eye changes occur naturally. It may therefore be hard to determine whether changes are caused by the treatment or not. But nothing is lost by looking out for visual changes whether degenerative or drug-induced.

The medicolegal consequences of drug induced visual loss may well be indefensible, and it is therefore sensible to obtain an ophthalmological opinion when symptoms present themselves in patients suffering from chronic systemic diseases.

The photographs of thyroid exophthalmos, diabetic retinopathy, and chloroquine retinopathy were reproduced by permission of the Institute of Ophthalmology; that of practolol-induced eye damage by kind permission of Mr Peter Wright.

# Appendix

Drugs that may have visual effects

| Drug | Blurring | Glaucoma | Retinal disease | Cataracts | Corneal and conjunctival damage |
|---|---|---|---|---|---|
| amitriptyline hydrochloride | S | + | | | |
| Anovlar (norethisterone, ethinyloestradiol) | T | | | | |
| Bellergal (belladonna, ergotamine, phenobarbitone) | S | + | | | |
| benzhexol hydrochloride | S | + | | | |
| betamethasone | S | + | | + | |
| biperiden lactate | S | + | | | |
| clomipramine hydrochloride | S | + | | | |
| chloramphenicol | S | | + | | |
| chloroquine phosphate | S | | + | | |
| chloroquine sulphate | S | | + | | |
| chlorpromazine hydrochloride | S | | | + | + |
| desipramine hydrochloride | S | + | | | |
| dicyclomine hydrochloride | S | + | | | |
| digitalis | | | + | | |
| digoxin | | | + | | |
| diphenhydramine hydrochloride | T | | | | |
| Donnatal (hyoscyamine, atropine, hyoscine, phenobarbitone) | S | + | | | |
| dothiepin hydrochloride | S | + | | | |
| emepronium bromide | S | + | | | |
| ethambutol | S | | + | | |
| ethopropazine hydrochloride | T | | | | |
| ethotoin | T | | | | |
| flavoxate hydrochloride | S | | + | | |
| glyceryl trinitrate | S | | + | | |
| glycopyrronium bromide | S | | + | | |
| imipramine | S | | + | | |
| indomethacin | T | | | + | |
| isocarboxazid | T | | | | |
| isopropamide iodide | S | + | | | |
| lanatoside C | T | | | | |
| levodopa | S | + | | | |
| Libraxin (clidinium, chlordiazepoxide) | S | + | | | |
| meprobamate | T | | | | |
| mepyramine maleate | T | | | | |
| metoprolol tartrate | T | | | | |
| methixene hydrochloride | S | + | | | |

| Drug | Blurring | Glaucoma | Retinal disease | Cataracts | Corneal and conjunctival damage |
|---|---|---|---|---|---|
| nalidixic acid | T | | | | |
| Neutradonna (aluminium sodium silicate, belladonna alkaloids) | S | + | | | |
| Norinyl (norethisterone, mestranol) | T | | | | |
| nortriptyline hydrochloride | S | + | | | |
| Orgraine (ergotamine tartrate, caffeine, hyoscyamine, atropine, phenacetin) | S | + | | | |
| orphenadrine citrate | S | + | | | |
| orphenadrine hydrochloride | S | + | | | |
| oxprenolol hydrochloride | T | | | | |
| pentaerythritol tetranitrate | S | + | | | |
| pentolinium tartrate | T | | | | |
| perphenazine | T | | | | |
| phenelzine sulphate | T | | | | |
| phenylpropanolamine hydrochloride | S | + | | | |
| phenytoin sodium | T | | | | |
| pipenzolate bromide | S | + | | | |
| poldine methylsulphate | S | + | | | |
| prednisolone sodium phosphate | S | + | | | |
| prochlorperazine mesylate | S | | | + | + |
| procyclidine hydrochloride | S | + | | | |
| promazine hydrochloride | T | | | | |
| propantheline bromide | S | + | | | |
| propranolol | T | | | | |
| protriptyline hydrochloride | S | + | | | |
| quinidine sulphate | T | | | | |
| quinine | | | + | | |
| sodium fusidate | T | | | | |
| thiethylperazine | S | | | + | + |
| thiopropazate hydrochloride | T | | | | |
| thioridazine hydrochloride | S | | + | | |
| tranylcypromine sulphate | T | | | | |
| trifluoperazine hydrochloride | S | | | + | |
| trimipramine maleate | S | + | | | |
| troxidone | S | + | | | |

S = Significant blurring. T = Transient blurring.